HELP!
MY MIND IS UNDER ATTACK

Replace Inner Chaos with Enduring Peace

MIKE MOORE

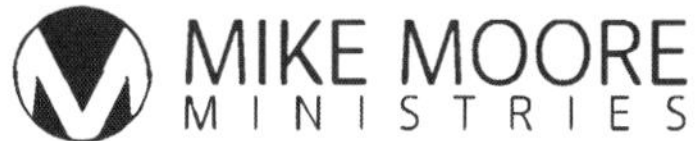

Help! My Mind is Under Attack: *Replace Inner Chaos with Enduring Peace*
By Mike Moore

©2022 Mike Moore | Printed in the United States of America

Paperback ISBN 978-1-7369777-1-2 / eBook ISBN 978-1-7369777-2-9

CONTENTS

GOOD MENTAL HEALTH IS ALREADY YOURS

When Jesus Christ died on the Cross, rose from the dead on the third day, and ascended to Heaven, He left us with a valuable gift. In John 14:27, Jesus said, "Peace I leave with you, My peace I give to you; not as the world gives do I give to you. Let not your heart be troubled, neither let it be afraid" (NKJV).

The Amplified Bible says, "Peace I leave with you; My [own] peace I now give *and* bequeath to you. Not as the world gives do I give to you. **Do not let** your hearts be troubled, neither let them be afraid. [**Stop allowing yourselves to be agitated and disturbed; and do not permit yourselves to be fearful and intimidated and cowardly and unsettled**]" (AMPC emphasis added). The Living Bible says, "I am leaving you with a gift—**peace of mind and heart! And the peace I give isn't fragile like the peace the world gives**. So don't be troubled or afraid" (TLB emphasis added). Jesus has given us a gift. We inherit that gift when we step into our position as members of His Kingdom.

Right away, we notice He says the peace He gave us is not like what the world gives. This peace...

- Passes all understanding (Philippians 4:7).
- Guards our hearts and minds (Philippians 4:7).
- Is anchored in Christ.

God's gift to you is good mental health. Another way to say that is, "The Prince of Peace (Isaiah 9:6) desires to give you *peace of mind*." How so? Consider this prayer that the Apostle John prayed over the saints in the early church.

> *"Beloved, I pray that you may prosper in all things and be in health, just as your **soul** prospers."* (3 John 2 NKJV)

The New English Translation of this verse says, "... I pray that all may go well with you and that you may be in good health, just as it is well with your soul." That should jog a familiar, musical hymn in your heart... *"It Is Well with My Soul."*

> *When peace like a river,*
> *attendeth my way,*
> *When sorrows like sea billows roll:*
> *Whatever my lot,*
> *Thou hast taught me to say,*
> *It is well,*
> *It is well with my soul.*

God's will for us as His children is to be well in our soul, which is our mind, will, and emotions. Our soul is where our mental health resides.

> *"'For I know the plans and thoughts that I have **for you**,'* says the LORD, **'plans for peace and well-being** *and not for disaster, to give you a future and a hope.'"* (Jeremiah 29:11 AMP)

He doesn't want us to be **troubled, agitated, or afraid** in our mind and emotions. This did not come from Him.

*"For God has not given us a spirit of fear, but of power and of love and of a **sound mind**."* (2 Timothy 1:7 NKJV emphasis added)

One of satan's main tactics is to attack us in our soul. The enemy...

- Understands the inseparable link between the mind and the body. Our body doesn't function apart from our mind.
- Knows that's where all sin starts.
- Seeks to distract Christians from their purpose.
- Attempts to uproot the Word of God you sowed in your heart, but he can't do it without your help.
- Thinks that if he can get you to believe a lie about God's Promises, you won't use your faith to claim those promises.
- Hopes if you think the armor of God doesn't work, you won't use it against him.
- Doesn't want you to resist him (James 4:7) because he would be obligated to have to flee from you.
- Knows **EVERYTHING** starts with a thought.

Throughout this book, you will be given godly truths to meditate on for renewing your mind. You will become better equipped to recognize satan's schemes for what they are, spoil his evil plans against you, take back control of your mental health, and begin walking out the wonderful plans God has in store for you.

It is well with your soul...

My prayer for you as you read is...

May God in Christ Jesus through the Holy Spirit, grant you the gift of mental health, emotional well-being, and physical healing in all things, in all ways, in all circumstances, so that you may prosper in the abundant life bestowed upon you through Christ Jesus, Amen.

CHAPTER 1

HELP! MY MIND IS UNDER ATTACK

*Finally, my brethren, be strong in the Lord and in the power of His might. Put on the **whole armor** of God, that you may be able to **stand against** the **wiles** of the **devil**.* (Ephesians 6:10-11 NKJV emphasis added)

Help my mind is under attack is the cry of many Christians. But knowing you are under attack and knowing how to overcome and gain the victory are two different things. The first issue is understanding the battlefield. Where is the war fought? The Bible reveals to us the mind is a combat zone. Secondly, we must understand who the enemy is, the strategies he uses, and why he's attacking our minds. Jesus said, the thief (devil) comes only to steal kill and destroy our lives. John 10:10 (NIV). Satan and his demon hosts study our lives looking for open doors and places whereby they can come in and begin to employ their "wiles." Satan then uses well-thought-out plans and strategies—the average Christian doesn't have a clue their enemy is using—to subtly attack their lives. Therefore, the average Christian is unprepared to stand against the wiles of the devil.

The enemy clutters our minds with millions of irrelevant, misleading, and lying thoughts. His strategy is to replace God's Word, His absolute and eternal truths, with lies from hell, the world, and the dark places or strongholds of our soul. There are thousands of pieces of orbiting space junk above Earth. Frequently, we hear of them crashing to the Earth or causing damage. Likewise, the destructive, dangerous junk entering our mind attacks, shatters, and tries to cause damage to our inner peace.

Standing Against the Wiles of the Devil

Ephesians 6:12 gives us two very important truths to be able to stand against our enemy. "For we wrestle **not** against flesh and blood, but against principalities, against powers, against the rulers of the darkness of this world, against spiritual wickedness in high places" (KJV emphasis added).

**All Christians are engaged in this war.
Our enemy is not our fellow man.**

We are not fighting against each other. Our battle is against principalities, powers, the rulers of the darkness of this world, and spiritual wickedness in heavenly places. In other words, our enemy is satan and his demon hosts. Therefore, we must learn what our weapons are and how to use them. Verse 13 begins our preparation for battle training, "Therefore, put on the complete armor of God, so that you will be able to [successfully] resist and **stand your ground** in the evil day [of danger], and having done everything [that the crisis demands], **to stand firm** [in your place, **fully prepared, immovable, victorious**]" (AMP emphasis added). It sounds to me like God wants us to stand because that's the position of victory. We're supposed to win. It's when we are flat on our backs that we are in trouble.

The Message Bible says, "Be prepared. You're up against far more than you can handle on your own. Take all the help you can get, every weapon God has issued, so that when it's all over but the shouting you'll still be on your feet. Truth, righteousness, peace, faith, and salvation are more than words. Learn how to apply them. You'll need them throughout your life. God's Word is an *indispensable weapon*" (MSG).

Ephesians 6:14-17 explains the different pieces of armor we are to put on in preparation for battle...

- *having girded your waist with truth [keeping your ammunition handy],*
- *having put on the breastplate of righteousness [knowing God's way],*
- *and having shod your feet with the preparation of the gospel of peace.*
- *Above all, taking the shield of faith with which you will be able to quench all the fiery darts of the wicked one.*
- *And take the helmet of salvation [to protect your mind],*
- *and the sword of the Spirit, which is the word of God"* (NKJV emphasis added).

Verse 16 says, "taking the shield of faith with which you will be able to quench all the fiery darts of the wicked one. The fiery darts represent a two-front attack. Satan attacks us with adverse circumstances stirring up disquieting fears and worries in our thoughts and feelings. God promises that with the shield of faith, we can quench and overcome adverse circumstances, and with the helmet of salvation we can protect our mind and our thoughts.

Satan Operates in the Mental Realm

The battlefield of the mind is where our biggest battle is going to be, not the flesh realm. There are five kinds of thoughts satan is going to throw our way. It is important we become familiar with his tactics so we can be prepared to battle against them.

1. Contradictory or Contrary Thoughts: Since the beginning of time, satan has attacked or attempted to attack the integrity of God. In other words, God says something in the Word, and satan hits us with a thought that contradicts that Word.

God says, "by His stripes you are healed," and satan hits you with a thought that you're sick and going to die.

God says, "I want you to forgive," and satan slides in with a thought about why you should be able to hold a grudge in this case.

God says, "you are worthy." God says, "you are fearfully and wonderfully made." God says, "you have the righteousness of God." Then satan comes and tells you how unworthy you are, that you are of low value, and that you cannot do things God's way.

God gives you a promise or God says something about you, and satan always comes with a thought that contradicts what God says.

2. Tormenting Thoughts: Tormenting thoughts are aimed at us personally. Satan hates us because we belong to God. Since he cannot get to God, he will attack us to try to hurt God. He loves to harass and agitate Christians.

3. Thoughts of Doubt: Thoughts of doubt are aimed at robbing us of God's blessings. When Peter was walking on the water, "he saw the wind *was* boisterous, he was afraid; and beginning to sink, he cried out, saying, 'Lord, save me!'" And Jesus said, "... why did you doubt?" (Matthew 14:30-31 NKJV).

4. Thoughts of Confusion: Satan understands we cannot be successful apart from wise decision-making, but we cannot make wise decisions if our mind is confused.

5. Thoughts of Failure: Thoughts of failure are aimed at getting us to quit.

If you learn how to shut satan out of your thought life, you shut down his operation.

---

2 Corinthians 11:3 says, "But I fear, lest by any means, as the serpent beguiled Eve through his subtilty, so your **minds** should be corrupted from the simplicity that is in Christ" (KJV emphasis added). The word *beguiled* means to deceive. The deception began in Eve's mind, her thought life. The Passion Translation says, "But now I'm afraid that just as Eve was deceived by the serpent's clever lies, **your thoughts may be corrupted** and you may lose your single-hearted devotion and pure love for Christ" (emphasis added). Satan gets Christians to backslide in the arena of their thought life—in their mind.

Satan blinds their minds to the Good News of the gospel of Christ.

*"But if our gospel be hid, it is hid to them that are lost in whom the god of this world hath **blinded the minds** of them which believe not, lest the light of the glorious gospel of Christ, who is the image of God, should shine unto them."*
(2 Corinthians 4:3-4 KJV emphasis added)

In my senior year in college, I was under conviction to become a Christian (to be saved), but my thinking was off. I thought God would just swoop down and save me without me giving Him permission. I said, "Lord, please don't save me my senior year. Don't mess up my senior year. We'll talk about this after." When I look back on that, I think how ridiculous that was, but my mind was blinded. I really wish I had gotten saved as a young child and was brought up in the things of God, but my mind was blinded.

Not only does satan blind our minds from the gospel, but he also programs us with his thoughts, with his ways, and with his information. In fact, our entire life before we make Jesus Lord, he is programming our minds.

When we accepted Jesus as our Lord and Savior, we were saved in our spirit, but our soul, which includes our mind, was not saved. It remained the same. Through God's Word, we can get our soul saved. That's going to be very important for us to remember because it is not automatic.

If you don't get your soul saved, even though you're born again and saved in your spirit, you could very well live out the program you received before you got saved and talk and act and walk just like a sinner. That is why some Christians struggle with worldliness.

Casting Down Imaginations

> *Though we walk in the flesh, **we do not war after the flesh**. (For the weapons of our warfare are not carnal but mighty through God to **the pulling down of strong holds**;) Casting down **imaginations**, and every high thing that exalteth itself against the knowledge of God, and bringing into captivity every thought to the obedience of Christ."* (2 Corinthians 10:3-5 KJV emphasis added)

This Scripture confirms we are engaged in a war. We walk in fleshly bodies, but when we war, we don't use our fleshly bodies to overcome the enemy because we are not fighting against flesh and blood. We cannot approach satan and demons the way we approach humans. We are warring in the mental arena.

> ***Stronghold*** {def}:
> A mindset, a way of thinking established over a period of time, fortified by custom, and resistant against change.

Remember, satan has not just been blinding our minds. He has been programming us to think a certain kind of way. He has been laying his mindset in us, brick by brick, thought by thought, and establishing strongholds in our minds.

Imagination {def}:
A mental picture, a deceptive fantasy

You cannot commit adultery without seeing yourself doing it first. You are created in such a way that you can't do anything without first seeing it in your mind. That's why when the field goal kicker gets on the open field, he mentally sees the football going through the goal. Satan understands that concept and brings mental pictures of a deceptive fantasy. He uses reasoning, an argument, a theory, speculation, and justification. God will tell you to do one thing, and satan will come and give you a reason why, in your case, you don't have to do it.

> *For though we walk (live) in the flesh, we are not carrying on our warfare according to the flesh and using mere human weapons. For the weapons of our warfare are not physical [weapons of flesh and blood], but they are **mighty before God for the overthrow and destruction of strongholds**, [Inasmuch as we] **refute arguments and theories and reasonings and every proud and lofty thing that sets itself up against the [true] knowledge of God**; and **we lead every thought and purpose away captive into the obedience of Christ** (the Messiah, the Anointed One).* (2 Corinthians 10:3-5 AMPC emphasis added)

The Bible says these things exalt themselves against God's Word. Our instructions are to cast these things down and "bring into captivity every thought." That implies these thoughts are rebel, outlaw thoughts, and we must arrest them. In other words, every thought that comes to our mind that does not come from God or conforms to His Word must be captured and taken captive.

**If the thought does not conform to God's Word,
the thought is from the enemy.**

The only way we can cast down an imagination and bring a thought into subjection is to know what God has to say. It's so unfortunate most Christians don't read their Bible enough to be able to measure their thoughts against the attacks satan brings into their minds. It makes it easy for satan to throw a thought at us when we have nothing to measure it by. This means **the more we know what it says in God's Word, the better we will be able to recognize the arguments and tactics satan is trying to use against us.**

Prepare Your Minds for Action

**So prepare your minds for action,
be completely sober [in spirit—steadfast,
self-disciplined, spiritually, and morally alert]...
(1 Peter 1:13 AMP)**

"Prepare your minds for action" is military language. When we go to war or we are in a war, do we send new recruits to the battlefield immediately after they enlist? No, of course not. We send them to boot camp for basic training to get them in shape for war. Once they get in shape, they can handle the pressures and attacks they will be facing when they engage the enemy.

Satan is out there. He is hitting us with thoughts every single day. He is relentless as he bombards our minds. 1 Peter 5:8 says, "Be on your guard and stay awake. Your enemy, the devil, is like a roaring lion, sneaking around to find someone to attack" (CEV). He's not coming to play with us. He's coming to destroy our lives. He wants to kill us. We need to be mentally awake. We must put our minds on high alert. We need to constantly be looking at the thoughts that come through our minds.

Satan understands that if our minds are off, it will affect our physical behavior. If our thoughts are wrong, we are going to have wrong behaviors. Romans 8:5 says, "Those who live according to the flesh [sinful nature] **have their minds set** on what the flesh [sinful nature] desires; those *who live in* accordance with the Spirit have their minds set on what the Spirit desires" (NIV emphasis added).

Galatians 5:19-21 reads, "The acts of the flesh [sinful nature] are obvious: sexual immorality, impurity, and debauchery; idolatry and witchcraft; hatred, discord, jealousy, fits of rage, selfish ambition, dissensions, factions and envy; drunkenness, orgies, and the like" (NIV emphasis added). In other words, satan appeals to this nature, and we begin to think about the things we picture our flesh would enjoy. That's when our physical behavior can be tempted to sin. The Bible says that our flesh enjoys those things; however, in the next verse, it mentions that our spirit enjoys love, joy, peace, longsuffering, kindness, goodness, faithfulness, gentleness, and self-control. The Bible here says those who are controlled by the flesh are those who are thinking on fleshly stuff.

Ephesians 2:2 says, "Wherein in time past ye walked according to the course of this world, according to the prince of the power of the air, the spirit that now worketh in the children of disobedience" (KJV). It's simply saying that when you were lost, you were controlled by the devil. The next verse says, "Among whom also we all had our conversation in times past in the lusts of our flesh **fulfilling the desires of the flesh and of the mind...**"

**Your thought life is directly linked to your behavior.
Control your thought life and you can control your behavior!**

Satan targets our minds because he understands the inseparable link between our thought life and our behavior. If we control our thought life, we can control our behavior. If we allow our thought life to run loose, our life will be loose.

Our biblical example is found in Mark 5:1-20. In this account, I want us to see in this extreme example how satan strives to manipulate a person's behavior through the mind. Jesus and the disciples met a man with an unclean spirit who had his dwelling among the tombs. He would cry out and cut himself with stones and he was naked. "When he saw Jesus from afar, he ran and worshiped Him. And he cried out with a loud voice and said, 'What have I to do with You, Jesus, Son of the Most High God? I implore You by God that You do not torment me.' For He said to him, 'Come out of the man, unclean spirit!'" (Verses 6-8 NKJV)

Jesus was talking to the evil spirit controlling this man. This man got in this shape because he didn't control his mind to the place where satan came in and took control of him. Satan wants to control us, too. If we do not control our thoughts, he may not possess us, but he will control areas of our lives, and we will be doing stuff and don't have a clue why. We will feel like we cannot help it.

Jesus asked the spirit, "What is your name?' And he answered, saying, 'My name is Legion: for we are many.'" Jesus cast the demons out of the man and sent them into swine (a herd of pigs). We can clearly see how the behavior of the swine was affected as soon as the evil spirits entered them. "And the herd ran violently down a steep place into the sea, and they were about two thousand, and were choked in the sea." Two thousand demons entered those 2,000 swine; they lost their minds, jumped in the water, and killed themselves.

It's possible to be in your right mind. Mark 5:14 describes the change in behavior of the man once the evil spirits left him and stopped tormenting his mind. "So those who fed the swine fled, and they told *it* in the city and in the country. And they went out to see what it was that had happened. Then they came to Jesus, and saw the one *who had been* demon-possessed and had the legion, sitting and clothed **and in his right mind**." Those spirits influenced that man through his mind. Notice how his behavior changed when he was in his right mind. I know that's an extreme case, but that is satan's tactic.

What's Influencing Your Thoughts?

In Matthew 16:21, Jesus began to explain to the disciples that He was going to go down to Jerusalem to be crucified, die, and on the third day He would be raised from the dead. In verse 22, Peter took Him aside and basically said, "No, you're not!" To his surprise, Jesus turned and looked at Peter and said, "Get behind Me, Satan! You are an offense to Me, for you are not mindful of the things of God, but the things of men" (NKJV). Peter is not demon-possessed, but at this point, Peter is yielding to the thoughts of the enemy. Satan is influencing his thoughts and Peter is acting on those thoughts.

In Luke 9:51-56, Jesus was getting ready to head to Jerusalem, but He was going to stop by a Samaritan village and conduct a meeting. James and John went ahead to prepare, but the people of Samaria said they did not want Jesus there. James and John got offended and went back to Jesus and, to paraphrase, said, "They don't want You in that city. Do You want us to call fire down from heaven, just like Elijah did, and burn them to a crisp?" Verses 55-56 says Jesus turned and rebuked them, and said, "You do not know what manner of spirit you are of. For the Son of Man did not come to destroy men's lives but to save *them*" (NKJV). They weren't demon-possessed, but at that point, they were being influenced in their thought life by satan.

Satan needs a yielded body to operate on the earth. The human body acts on information or directions given through the mind.

Satan's attack will begin in the mind. Whatever the mind continually thinks on, the body will eventually respond to.

Genesis 6:4-5 gives us another biblical example. "There were giants in the earth in those days; and also after that, when the sons of God came in unto the daughters of men, and they bare children to them, the same became mighty men which were of old, men of renown. And God saw that the wickedness of man was great in the earth, and that **every imagination of the thoughts of his heart [mind] was only evil continually**" (KJV emphasis added).

The Thought Precedes the Act

In Matthew 5:27-28, Jesus explained this concept to His followers by using adultery as an example. "Ye have heard that it was said by them of old time, Thou shalt not commit adultery, but I say unto you, that whosoever looketh on a woman to lust after her **hath committed adultery with her already in his heart [mind]**" (KJV emphasis added). He's literally saying that adultery, which is an act—a behavior—doesn't begin in the bedroom. It doesn't begin with the physical action. He says it begins in a person's thought life. One can't commit adultery without first thinking about it.

Matthew 15:19 says, "For out of the heart proceed evil thoughts, murders, adulteries, fornications, thefts, false witness, blasphemies" (KJV).

Notice how the thought precedes the act: Jesus reveals that...

- murder begins with an evil thought.
- adultery begins with an evil thought.
- fornication begins with an evil thought.
- stealing begins with an evil thought.
- lying begins with an evil thought.

›› ASK YOURSELF...

Have I had thoughts that are contrary to God's Word?
How can I shut down satan's operation?

›› APPLY WHAT YOU'VE LEARNED

Prepare your mind for action by reviewing the tactics satan may use to mess with your thoughts. The best way to prepare is to study God's Word. Choose a recent tactic satan has used against you. Find a Scripture that contradicts satan's attack and confess it. When a thought that goes against what God says comes to your mind, replace it with God's Word. Repetition is the key to learning, so keep doing this until it becomes a habit to you.

CHAPTER 2

REBUKE THE SATANIC PATTERN

To keep Satan from getting the advantage over us; for ***we are not ignorant of his wiles and intentions***. (2 Corinthians 2:11 AMPC emphasis added)

We have begun to learn satan's tactics to try and use our minds to influence our behavior. Next, we need to learn about the weapons he uses, as well as how to defend ourselves and go on the offensive to gain victory.

Satan's main weaponry consists of lies and deception.

Satan is the father of lies. He is the originator of lying. In fact, when speaking with His critics who resisted His teachings, Jesus said in John 8:44...

"You belong to your father, the devil, and you want to carry out your father's desires. He was a murderer from the beginning, not holding to the truth, for ***there is no truth in him***. *When he lies, he speaks his native language, for* ***he is a liar and the father of lies***.*"* (NIV emphasis added)

*"You are just like your true father, the devil; and you spend your time pursuing the things your father loves. **He started out as a killer, and he cannot tolerate truth because he is void of anything true. At the core of his character, he is a liar**; everything he speaks originates in these lies because he is the father of lies"* (VOICE emphasis added).

Satan is a liar and a deceiver. Deception is when satan has successfully canceled out tomorrow's consequences by emphasizing today's delight in our mind or in our thinking. 2 Corinthians 2:11 warns, "After all, we don't want to unwittingly give Satan an opening for yet more mischief—we're not oblivious to his sly ways!" (MSG). In other words, we do not have to be ignorant of satan's strategies and patterns. So then, why are many in the Body of Christ getting beat at the game of life?

Evil is on the earth because Lucifer had already rebelled. He, as a fallen angel, had already been cast out of heaven onto the earth. There was no evil on earth before Lucifer became satan and lost his place in heaven. He became the father of evil, lies, and deception. His sole purpose then became to kill, steal, and destroy man in order to hurt God.

Enter the Father of Lies and Deception (Genesis 3:1-7 NKJV – emphasis and commentary added)

*Now the serpent was more cunning than any beast of the field which the Lord God had made. And he said to the woman, **"Has God indeed said**, 'You shall not eat of every tree of the garden'?"*

[Satan Strategy: He tries to sow a seed of doubt in the mind.]

And the woman said to the serpent, "We may eat the fruit of the trees of the garden; but of the fruit of the tree which is in the midst of the garden, God has said, 'You shall not eat it, nor shall you touch it, lest you die.'"

*Then the serpent said to the woman, **"You will not surely die.** For God knows that in the day you eat of it your eyes will be opened, and you will be like God, knowing good and evil."*

So when the woman saw [Satan Strategy: He got her to imagine] *that the tree was good for food, that it was pleasant to the eyes, and a tree desirable to make one wise, **she took of its fruit and ate.*** [Satan Strategy: He wanted her to act on what she imagined.] *She also gave to her husband with her, and he ate. Then the eyes of both of them were opened, and they knew that they were naked; and they sewed fig leaves together and made themselves coverings.*

The Repercussions of Listening to the Father of Lies and Deception (Genesis 3:8-13 NKJV)

And they heard the sound of the LORD God walking in the garden in the cool of the day, and Adam and his wife hid themselves from the presence of the LORD God among the trees of the garden.

Then the LORD God called to Adam and said to him, "Where are you?"

So he said, "I heard Your voice in the garden, and I was afraid because I was naked; and I hid myself."

And He said, "Who told you that you were naked? Have you eaten from the tree of which I commanded you that you should not eat?"

Then the man said, "The woman whom You gave to be with

me, she gave me of the tree, and I ate."

And the Lord *God said to the woman, "What is this you have done?" The woman said, "The serpent deceived me, and I ate."*

**Therefore the Lord God sent him out of the garden of
Eden to till the ground from which he was taken.
So He [God] drove out the man;
and He placed cherubim at the east of the garden of
Eden, and a flaming sword which turned every way, to
guard the way to the tree of life. (Genesis 3:23-24)**

The tree Adam was told not to eat from was not the tree of evil. It was not the tree of good. It was the tree of the knowledge of good and evil. This implies that at this point, man only knew good. It was God's will Adam not to know the other side. God told Adam, "Don't eat from that because if you eat from that, you'll come into the experience of what evil is. I don't want you to experience that. If you eat from it, you are going to die."

God said, "Of every tree you may eat" before He said don't eat of this one tree. Our problem is we don't understand that whenever God says "DON'T" to something, He's saying "DO" to something else. Whenever God says "YOU CAN'T" to one thing, He's saying "YOU CAN" to something else.

Genesis 3:1 says, "Now the serpent was more crafty than any of the wild animals the Lord God had made. He said to the woman, "Did God **really** say, 'You must not eat from any tree in the garden'" (NIV emphasis added)?

Satan is asking a question. He's engaging in a conversation. Our problem here is we need to learn we must not engage in a conversation with the devil. Eve gave attention to the subtle, smart, cunning, conniving, deceptive, crafty, and underhanded devil disguised as a "serpent."

He won't say, "I am the devil. I am trying to trick you." That's not his pattern.

When he sends a thought into our mind, we should ignore him. However, the problem here is that when he asked her a question, she entered into a dialogue with him. **She entertained the thought.**

"And the woman said to the serpent, 'We may eat the fruit of the trees of the garden; but of the fruit of the tree which *is* in the midst of the garden,' God has said, 'You shall not eat it, nor shall you touch it, lest you die.' Then the serpent said to the woman, 'You will not surely die'" (NKJV). This was a contradictory or contrary thought. God said, "You're going to die," and the devil said, "No, you're not." Satan is still saying the same thing. It is part of the satanic pattern.

The next step in this satanic pattern is to introduce a mental picture to her imagination. It was a deceptive fantasy, a reasoning, an argument, a justification to tempt her into an action. He said, "No, you're not going to die, and here's the reason." In other words, here's the argument. Here's the imagination. Here's why it's all right in your case. He is still saying the same thing. It's all right in your case because your situation is different.

In verse 4-5, the serpent said to the woman, "You will not surely die. For God knows that in the day you eat of it your eyes will be opened, and you will be like God, knowing good and evil." Notice what satan did. He made God the problem.

Adam and Eve were given the perfect life, the perfect environment, and everything was good, but they lost all the benefits of walking with God. They are now on the outside looking back at what they have lost.

Ask Yourself...

If they could have seen this repercussion from the beginning, do you think they would have listened to satan's lies and made the same mistake?

No, of course not. They didn't see the end. **The satanic pattern is to never show us the end. He shows us the beginning and the immediate benefit of a certain behavior or choice. That's how he functions.**

God is totally different. God will show us the beginning and the end right up front. He'll say, "If you do this, I'll bless you and if you don't do this, you're going to be cursed." In Genesis 2:16, the Lord God commanded the man, saying, "Of every tree of the garden you freely eat; but of the tree of the knowledge of good and evil you shall not eat, for in the day that you eat of it you shall surely die'" (NKJV).

God says, "Here's what I want for you. I am on your side. I am the creator. I'm the giver of all life and all that is good. All I want you to experience is good. However, because I want you to love Me the way I love you, you must have a chance to choose. I don't want robots. I don't want people to just obey Me because they have to. Love is a choice."

You can choose God, or you can choose the devil. Trying to listen to both makes you double-minded.

The satanic pattern is to make God the "bad guy." He says, "Let me tell you why God doesn't want you to eat from that tree. He just doesn't want you to have any fun. He just wants you to miss out on everything. You've got a right to have some fun. He's just trying to hold out on you. He doesn't want you to have a life. God just wants you to be religious while everybody else is having fun. God is the problem."

Remember we are to cast down imaginations. This imagination is an argument. It's a reason (justification) why you can do what God says you shouldn't do. However, the Bible says whenever God says something and anything comes to your mind that contradicts what God says and then gives you a reason or a justification or an argument why it's all right for you, it is an **outlaw rebel thought** and is exalting itself against the knowledge of God. You better capture that thought and bring it under control.

The Satanic Pattern:
1. **A contradictory thought is introduced.**
2. **Followed by an argument, a justification, or a reason.**
3. **If the thought is not dealt with properly, you end up with a deceptive fantasy.**

First, the serpent said to the woman, "You will not surely die." That's the contradictory thought.

Second, "For God knows that in the day you eat of it your eyes will be opened, and you will be like God, knowing good and evil." That's the argument, the reason, the justification.

The deceptive fantasy shows up in verse 6, "So when the woman saw that the tree *was* good for food, that it *was* pleasant to the eyes, and a tree desirable to make *one* wise, she took of its fruit and ate. She also gave to her husband with her, and he ate."

What did the woman see?

**The mental picture satan painted for her said,
the tree was good for food;
the fruit was pleasant to the eyes;
and it was desirable.**

She saw all this and had never tasted its fruit, so how did she know it was good and pleasant?

**She did not cast down the imagination!
When satan painted an enticing picture in her mind,
she also saw how it would make her wise.**

What happened after she saw it in her mind?

She acted on that deceptive fantasy.

She took the fruit.
She ate the fruit.
She even gave some to her husband.

It was a deceptive fantasy that caused her to forget God said she would die if she ate of it.

Satan Perverts What God Says

Satan's goal is to have us believe and imagine the reverse of what God intended. What God intended is for us to do is hear what He says and act on His truth. We are to cast down any imagination, perception or thought that exalts itself against the knowledge of what God has said. We are supposed to meditate on and develop a mental picture of what God says we should do because the act will always follow the thought. What God says is always for our good.

Satan threw contradiction and argument—based on lies, deception, and a perversion of God's truth—at Eve. Then he set up a deceptive picture of beauty making God out to be the bad guy. He's still doing the same thing, using the same tactic, and implementing the same satanic pattern.

Satan always contradicts what God says: God said, "we will die if we do this," but satan said, "no you won't." After he contradicts what God says, satan gives us an argument or a reason or a justification why our "special case" it's all right to do what God said not to do. If we don't deal with that argument properly, cast down that imagination, we will end up with a deceptive fantasy where suddenly we see beauty in what God says is not good.

Look what happened to Adam and Eve. They are now outside the Garden and realizing what they have lost. Now, they can see clearly and experiencing regret. That's where we are going to be every time we disobey God. We are going to be on the outside of the blessing God had for us.

When it's all said and done, satan will pull the covers back to show us the consequences of our choice and we will feel like fools for not doing things God's way.

›› ASK YOURSELF...

Have I been deceived by the father of lies?

Describe it:
What were the consequences?

What can I do to avoid being deceived again?

›› APPLY WHAT YOU'VE LEARNED

Let's put what you've learned into practice. <u>Satan's GOAL is to attack your mental health</u>. **To counteract the Satanic Pattern,** make spending time with God and finding out what He says about things a priority. Dedicate a specific amount of time each day to do this. For example, this could include reading God's Word, praying, meditating, listening to podcasts, reading articles, etc.

If there is a specific area (e.g., sickness, rejection, insecurity) where satan is attacking you, focus your time on reading, praying, and/or meditating in that area.

CHAPTER 3

STOP WORRYING

I will now provide you with multiple biblical definitions of *worry* so we can know what it is and recognize it. If we don't understand it, we could very well think that worrying is normal. In fact, we could even go further and think that worry is a friend. If we think worry is normal, then we will tolerate, embrace, and accept it. If we think worry is a friend, we will invite it to dinner and fellowship with it. However, if we discover that it is an enemy to our peace and our mental health, there's a good chance we will shut the door and resist it.

What Is Worry?

- To be anxious, uptight
- To be full of care ("to take thought")
- Concern over the future regarding something you cannot do anything about right now (i.e., borrowing on tomorrow's problems today)
- To divide, part, rip, or tear; to divide the mind or be drawn in different directions
- Mental distress
- Thinking the worst
- To choke or strangle the mind

- To be distracted
- To have a troubling concern
- Placing more confidence in your circumstances than trusting God and His Word
- Wasted or misguided mental energy
- Meditation on the lies of the devil

Worry and anxiety are connected to fear. Fear of something bad happening in the future. Fear of not having enough resources. Fear of failure. Common things people worry about include their finances (paying bills), job security, safety, their family, their health, acceptance from others, work expectations, their own abilities, and more. However, notice the command given in Philippians 4:6.

> *"Be careful for nothing..."* (KJV)
> *"Do not be anxious or worried about anything..."*(AMP)
> *"Be anxious for nothing..."* (NKJV)

Scripture indicates there is no legitimate reason to be concerned, worried, or anxious about anything in your life. God is a loving God. He would never command us to do something that we are unable to do. Therefore, if He is saying not to worry, that means it is within our power to do so. To not do so would be sin.

> *"Therefore I [Jesus] say to you, **do not worry about your life,** what you will eat or what you will drink; nor about your body, what you will put on. Is not life more than food and the body more than clothing? Look at the birds of the air, for they neither sow nor reap nor gather into barns; **yet your heavenly Father** feeds them. Are you not of more value than they? Which of you by **worrying** can add one cubit to his stature?*
>
> *So **why do you worry** about clothing? Consider the lilies of the field, how they grow: they neither toil nor spin; and*

*yet I say to you that even Solomon in all his glory was not arrayed like one of these. Now if God so clothes the grass of the field, which today is, and tomorrow is thrown into the oven, will He not much more clothe you, **O you of little faith**?*

*Therefore **do not worry, saying,** 'What shall we eat?' or 'What shall we drink?' or 'What shall we wear?' For after all these things the Gentiles seek. **For your heavenly Father knows that you need all these things.** But seek first the kingdom of God and His righteousness, and all these things shall be added to you. Therefore **do not worry about tomorrow, for tomorrow will worry about its own things**. Sufficient for the day is its own trouble."* (Matthew 6:25-34 NKJV emphasis added)

Get your focus right. Jesus is assuring you… you can go through life without worrying.

The King James Version says to "take no thought for your life." Therefore, if we "take thought" and worry about all those things, we are disobeying Jesus. Jesus is saying that if God gave us life, won't He also make sure that we have the things we need to continue living? If we are worried about what we eat, what we drink, what we put on, our utilities, bills, car notes, and all that stuff, it is because we have the wrong focus.

What's So Bad About Worrying?

Jesus said, "Oh, you of little faith." Worry is *a blatant distrust of the power and love of God.* Worry is an affront and an insult to God. It's an affront to God's ability and to His willingness to do something about our problem. We're saying to God, "You can't handle my problem. My problem is too big for You, or I am not important enough to You." It is disrespectful to His power, His ability, His love, and His willingness to handle our problem.

Worry is basically taking ownership of the problem and declaring yourself bigger than God because you believe and act like God can't handle it.

In verse 26, Jesus says, "Look at the birds of the air, for they neither sow nor reap nor gather into barns; **yet your heavenly Father** feeds them. Are you not of more value than they?" For the most part, children don't worry. We never see kids getting up in the morning and asking us, "Did you pay the mortgage this month?" Have you seen them going through the bills to see what still needs to be paid? They are just footloose and fancy-free. They don't worry about whether there is food for them unless they've experienced a lack. Very seldom do we see children get ulcers. For the most part, kids don't worry about it because they **trust** daddy or mommy to handle it. They don't even care to know the details of how things got paid.

Worry *is also distrust in God's faithfulness to do what He said He would do.* If we say things like, "I know the Bible says it, but...," that's an insult to God because we're saying we can't trust God to do what He says He will do. Imagine if our child said, "I know mommy said, but..."

Worry is like a slap in the face of God!

In verse 32 we read, "For after all these things, **do the Gentiles seek for your heavenly father, knoweth that you have need of all these things**" (KJV). This ties in with Ephesians 2:11-12 where Paul says, "Therefore remember that you, once Gentiles in the flesh— who are called Uncircumcision by what is called the Circumcision made in the flesh by hands—that at that time you were without Christ, being aliens from the commonwealth of Israel and strangers from the covenants of promise, having no hope and without God in the world" (NKJV). In other words, before we knew Jesus, we were strangers from the covenant of promise, having no hope, and without God. Another word for Gentiles could be *orphans* or *sinners*. He says Gentiles—orphans or sinners—seek these things because they do not have hope without God.

> *But seek ye first the kingdom of God, and his righteousness; and all these things shall be added unto you. Take therefore no thought for the morrow: for the morrow shall take thought for the things of itself. Sufficient unto the day is the evil thereof.* (Matthew 6:33-34 KJV)

Do not seek the things the Gentile seek. An orphan doesn't have a father or mother, so the orphan must scrounge around on his or her own. **We are not orphans.** Remember, Gentiles or sinners don't have a covenant because they are without God and without hope in the world. They have to seek these things on their own, but we are not without God. We're not without a covenant.

Remember, we are not without a father. Jesus promised, "I will not leave you orphans; I will come to you" (John 14:18 NKJV). Our Heavenly Father knows we have need of all these things. When we seek things and then worry, we are acting out of character. We are acting like an orphan. We're acting like a person who doesn't have a daddy who knows we need these things. Jesus says, "Seek first the kingdom" (God's way of doing things) and everything else will come. However, we must trust Him.

Keys to Overcoming Worry

Jesus begins to give us keys to dealing with worry in Matthew 6:31. *"Therefore, **take no thought, saying**, What shall we eat? or, What shall we drink? or, Wherewithal shall we be clothed" (KJV)?* There are two keys here to overcoming worry:

1. Control our thoughts.
2. Control our words.

Key #1: Control Our Thoughts

What Jesus is saying is that satan is going to bring thoughts to our mind. The mind is the major battleground we face. There will never be a place in our Christian experience where satan will not have access to our mind. That's the place where he comes to try to control our life. He attacks us in our thoughts. He always tries to bring us thoughts of lack, some form of loss, some thought of failure, some inability to make it, that some bills won't be paid, and won't have enough money for our children to go to college.

"Therefore, take no thought," which means when those thoughts come, **don't take them!** Not every thought that comes to our mind is from God. If we don't learn how to take control of our thoughts, the thoughts from satan (those that don't align with God's Word) will turn into strongholds (fortified mindsets). If we don't control our thoughts, we will develop a mental picture of defeat.

One of the college students in our ministry asked me, "Have you ever gone into a test knowing you were going to fail?" I said, "I never had that experience." If we go into a test fearing failure, we have allowed satan to build a mental image of failure in our mind. The Bible instructs us to "cast down imaginations." The root word for imaginations is *image*. Satan tries to erect a picture or image of failure in our mind, and then he uses circumstances to create that image. Remember, one of the definitions of worry was "placing more confidence in our circumstances than trusting God and His Word." That's how we know God's Word has departed from our eyes. We are looking at the circumstances instead of God because satan has begun to erect an image in our mind, but that's not the end of it. It still won't harm us unless we declare it.

Key #2: Control Our Words

A thought unspoken will die unborn.

Let's look back at verse 31, **"Therefore take no thought, saying,** What shall we eat? or, What shall we drink? or, Wherewithal shall we be clothed?" (KJV).

If we say it, then we are giving life to it. Proverbs 18:21a says, "Death and life are in the power of the tongue" (KJV). We can tell when satan is winning when we speak the negative thought. When we speak that thought, we give life to it. That's exactly what the enemy wants. That's why he's building that image in our mind. He's trying to instill fear in us. Worry and anxiety are connected to fear. When we talk about our fears, we build an image, and we enlarge the problem in our mind. When we talk about our faith, we enlarge God in our mind.

In Luke 12, Jesus was talking about seeking first the kingdom of God, then He says in verse 32, **"fear not,** little flock; it is your father's good pleasure to give you the kingdom" (KJV). He said don't be afraid. Well, where did the fear come from? It came from looking at our circumstances and satan building a mental image of failure.

Whether it's academics, marriage, dating, parenting, finances, or health on any level, satan must first build a mental picture. Once we see it, the Word says for **us** to cast it down. Nobody can do this for us.

I used to see myself failing...
I saw myself as poor...
I felt poor...
I thought poor, and...
I had a mental image of poverty...

There are people who get married with the expectation it will fail, although there are no outward reasons to support their view. They begin to express their fears about things that could go wrong.

"My spouse is probably going to cheat on me."
"My spouse will get bored with me."
"This probably won't last."

A common fear is public speaking. Some people <u>see</u> themselves trembling in front of others <u>before</u> they've even reached the stage or the meeting to give the presentation. They don't see themselves standing in front of a crowd and expressing their hearts to others. Their fears come out in their self-talk and conversations with others.

"I'm not a speaker."
"I'm not comfortable speaking in front of folks."
"What if no one listens?"
"They're going to laugh at me."

What they've done is given life to the mental image satan has built in their minds. The more they confess it, the more they believe it. However, the truth is God did not create us that way. God created us to be communicators. That is why Jesus said we are to go into all the world and preach the gospel. How can we go into all the world and preach the gospel if we can't talk to people? How in the world can we obey the great commission if we are afraid of failure or persecution? Satan built a mental picture of failure in some of our minds.

Many people speak their negative thinking when they are looking for a new job. Before they contact the company, some will say...

"They are probably not even hiring."
"Even if I get an interview, I'm sure I won't get the job."
"I'm sure there are more qualified candidates."

How does saying these things to ourselves or others benefit us?

2 Corinthians 10:3-4 declares, "For though we walk in the flesh, we do not war after the flesh. For the weapons of our warfare are not carnal, but mighty through God to the pulling down of strongholds"

(KJV). That's a thought stronghold, an inferior way of thinking, or a negative and destructive mindset. Satan's built up something in our mind using thoughts.

Paul goes on to say, "Casting down imaginations." In this case, it's a mental picture of failure. We are told to cast down imaginations "and every high thing that exalteth itself against the knowledge of God, and **bringing into captivity every thought** to the obedience of Christ" (KJV). That's good news because this means **we** are in control of our thought life! Remember self-control (temperance) is a fruit of the Spirit.

The devil is only in control of our thought life if we let him be in control.

Proverbs 30:32 gives us practical advice. It says, "If you have been foolish in exalting yourself, or if you have devised evil, *put your* hand on *your* mouth" (NKJV). The reason he says to put our hand on our mouth is because if we don't speak it out, it will die. The Bible says, "Death and life are in the power of the tongue: **and they that love it shall eat the fruit thereof**" (Proverbs 18:21 KJV emphasis added). When we speak our weakness, we give life to our weakness. When we speak about our inability, the result is we'll eat the fruit of our inabilities. Let the thought die by not vocalizing it!

Be Present

Matthew 6:34 says, "Therefore **do not worry about tomorrow, for tomorrow will worry about its own things**. Sufficient for the day is its own trouble" (NKJV emphasis added). Live one day at a time. He's not saying it's wrong to plan. He's not talking against foresight, but don't live in the past, and don't live in the future. Don't get caught up in worrying about tomorrow. We should live in the present moment and plan for the future, rather than worrying about it.

Don't live in the past. Don't live in the future.
In the present, God is present.
He is God of the NOW!

"If you are depressed, you are living in the past.
If you are anxious, you are living in the future.
If you are at peace, you are living in the present."
-Anonymous[1]

If we will do what we need to do today, tomorrow will be good. That's true on any level. If we do what we need to do today about our life spiritually, we will have a good life spiritually tomorrow. If we do what we need to do physically and eat right, rest our body, and do everything we should, we don't have to worry about our tomorrow, our tomorrow will be good. If we do what's right regarding our spouse and our children, we don't have to worry about them down the road.

Here's something to consider. "Research over the last 20 years has shown that preventable factors—factors amenable to change—could account for 40 percent or more of premature deaths."[2] If we could make changes that would involve not smoking or drinking alcohol, avoiding overeating, staying physically fit, reducing stress and worry, eating nutritiously, etc., we would have mental and physical health. We would prosper and live longer. So...

Just do what you need to do today.
If you do what you need to do today,
it'll be fine tomorrow.

---

1 Motivational Quotes (12938 quotes) (goodreads.com)

2 https://www.ncbi.nlm.nih.gov/books/NBK279981/

We can choose not to worry about the future, but will we? Trust Jesus' admonition, "Don't worry." Our mental health depends on it.

›› ASK YOURSELF...

What do I find myself worrying about most often?
When I worry, what have I tried to do to stop it?
Am I controlling my thoughts?
Do I talk about my fears or my faith?

›› APPLY WHAT YOU'VE LEARNED

Start a dialogue with God by praying this prayer. Allow Him to help you with your feelings of worry and anxiety. You don't have to do it alone. Remember, you're not an orphan. Invite Him into your situation.

Father God, I know that You care for me and that you care about every detail of my life. Help me to find comfort and rest in that. I ask You by the power of Your Spirit to help me to live one day at a time, to not worry about tomorrow but instead focus on what you're doing in my life right now. Help me to trust in Your promise to take care of every one of my needs — financial, relational, physical, social, spiritual, and emotional. Help me to trust you more and resist the urge to worry or be anxious.

I pray in Jesus' Name. Amen.

CHAPTER 4

ERADICATE WORRY FROM YOUR LIFE

The Bible teaches it is possible to live a worry-free life. The Apostle Paul has given us simple, yet profound, instructions on how to eradicate worry. Remember in Philippians 4:6 he says, "Do not be anxious or worried about anything" (AMP). I believe we can all do it. However, first we need to understand how God wants us to handle the challenges of life. At that point, we can take the principles (learning what God says about a matter) and apply them not only to worry, but to stress, depression, rejection, and more.

*"Why do you call Me, 'Lord, Lord,' and **do not practice** what I tell you? Everyone who comes to Me and listens to My words **and obeys** them, I will show you whom he is like: he is like a [far-sighted, practical, and sensible] man building a house, who dug deep and laid a foundation on the rock; and when a flood occurred, the torrent burst against that house and yet could not shake it, because it had been securely built and founded on the rock.*

*But the one who has **[merely] heard and has not practiced [what I say]**, is like a [foolish] man who built a house on the ground without any foundation, and the torrent burst* *against it; and it immediately collapsed, and the ruin of that house was great." (Luke 6:46-49 AMP emphasis added)*

We have a definition of obedience here. The Bible says two men built houses. One house stood against the storm, and one house collapsed against the storm. Maybe the difference was that one person was saved and the other person was not saved. Well, that can't be the difference because Christians are devastated every day by challenges, problems, and situations. There must be more to it. Maybe one Christian was a member of a church, and the other Christian really was just kind of floating around. Is that the difference? No, Jesus said they needed to listen and then obey **by doing** what He told them to do.

> *But **prove yourselves doers of the word** [actively and continually obeying God's precepts], **and not merely listeners** [who hear the word but fail to internalize its meaning], **deluding yourselves** [by unsound reasoning contrary to the truth]. For if anyone only listens to the word without obeying it, he is like a man who looks very carefully at his natural face in a mirror; for once he has looked at himself and gone away, he immediately forgets what he looked like. But he who looks carefully into the perfect law, the law of liberty, and **faithfully abides by it**, not having become a [careless] listener who forgets but **an active doer** [who obeys], **he will be blessed and favored by God in what he does [in his life of obedience].** (James 1:22-25 AMP emphasis added)*

The Bible describes those who hear the Word of God, but they are not doers of the Word. Once they leave, they forget not only what they have heard, but also who they are. We cannot forget who we are. Otherwise, when the challenges, the problems, or the circumstances come, we can't apply or be doers of the Word.

**The Bible declares a man is blessed when he
takes the instructions he has received,
does what they tell him to do,
and lives his life by the Word.**

The Sources of Worry and Anxiety Pressure

Even though God said don't worry, the first thing we must understand about overcoming is simply this: worrisome thoughts and situations will come our way. We're going to experience pressure from three different sources. The first source is identified in the Parable of the Sower in Mark 4:14-19.

*The sower sows the word [of God, the good news regarding the way of salvation]. These [in the first group] are the ones along the road where the word is sown; but when they hear, **Satan** immediately comes and takes away the word which has been sown in them.*

*In a similar way these [in the second group] are the ones on whom seed was sown on rocky ground, who, when they hear the word, immediately receive it with joy [but accept it only superficially]; and they have no real root in themselves, so they endure only for a little while; then, **when trouble or persecution comes because of the word,** immediately they [are offended and displeased at being associated with Me and] stumble and fall away.*

*And others are the ones on whom seed was sown among the thorns; these are the ones who have heard the word, but the **worries and cares of the world** [the distractions of this age with its worldly pleasures], and the deceitfulness [and the false security or glamour] of wealth [or fame], and the passionate desires for all the other things*

creep in and choke out the word, and it becomes unfruitful.
(AMP emphasis added)

1. Satan pressures us with worry.

In the Parable of the Sower, Jesus reveals that satan makes it his job to attempt to cause the seed of the Word to not produce in our lives. He uses affliction (pain and suffering), persecution, lust for other things, the deceitfulness of riches, and the **worries and cares of the world**. It only mentions satan at the beginning of this passage, but even though we don't see him anymore, he's behind the others, causing the pressure of circumstances. He is behind the trouble, persecution, the lust for other things, and the deceitfulness of riches. The enemy is also instigating the cares of this world. Satan will always tempt us to worry.

Pressure from satan is continual and relentless because he understands if he can get us to worry, the Word can't produce blessings and abundance in our life. That's his goal. He may press us to sin, which causes us not to produce. He'll also take a legitimate concern like a loved one being ill. Their illness becomes a distraction and begins pulling us in all different directions as their caregiver. We now tell ourselves we "**don't have time** to be in the Word and do what it says to do." Satan has now successfully used the cares of our life to keep the Word from producing fruit in our life. When any care of the world distracts us, recognize it for what it is: a satanic tactic. No matter how legitimate the reason appears, immediately seek God by praising Him, praying, and giving thanks, not for the situation, but because of who He is. (I'll get more into prayer and thanksgiving a little later.)

2. People pressure us to worry.

The second source of pressure is found in Mark 4:37-38. "And a fierce windstorm began to blow, and waves were breaking over the boat, so that it was already being swamped. But Jesus was in the stern, asleep [with His head] on the [sailor's leather] cushion. And they woke Him and said to Him, 'Teacher, do You not care that we are about to die?'" (AMP).

We're going to feel pressure from people. It's a strange thing, but misery loves company. There are Christians who will get angry when we start operating in this carefree lifestyle, where we're not worried about anything. When we're not worrying and up-in-arms about a situation like they are, they'll interpret it as not caring and a lack of concern. This is because worrying is a normal response in society. We'll appear strange (as the Bible says, a "peculiar people") because we have transferred ownership of the problem over to the Lord and have let the Lord own the problem.

3. *Our flesh pressures us to worry.*

We will feel pressure from **our own flesh** because it's normal for our flesh to want to worry. In fact, it takes discipline **not** to worry. **We** must make the choice not to worry. If we don't make the choice, God can't do it for us. That's the decision each one of us must make because our spouse can't make it, our parents can't make it, our friends can't make it, and our pastor can't make it for us.

We choose to agree with the truths of Scripture. When we offer the excuse, *I cannot help but worry*, we're saying God is being unfair by asking us to do something we cannot do. The very fact He says *don't worry about anything* means there's grace available to either do it or not do it.

**God gives us the grace
to not worry. Ask for it.**
Lord, set me free from worry!

How to Conquer Worry

The Word of God in Philippians 4:6-9 (AMP) is literally the answer. It gives us a step-by-step guide to being free from worry and anxiety. Let's first review the entire passage, and then we'll unpack each solution to bring clarity.

> ***Do not be anxious or worried about anything***, *but in everything [**every circumstance** and situation] by **prayer***

and petition with thanksgiving, continue to make your [specific] requests known to God. And the peace of God [that peace which reassures the heart, that peace] which transcends all understanding, [that peace which] stands guard over your hearts and your minds in Christ Jesus [is yours].

*Finally, believers, whatever is true, whatever is honorable and worthy of respect, whatever is right and confirmed by God's word, whatever is pure and wholesome, whatever is lovely and brings peace, whatever is admirable and of good repute; if there is any excellence, if there is anything worthy of praise, **think continually on these things** [center your mind on them, and implant them in your heart]. The things which you have learned and received and heard and seen in me, **practice these things [in daily life]**, and the **God [who is the source] of peace and well-being** will be with you.* (Philippians 4:6-9 AMP emphasis added)

Four Steps to Conquering Worry

1. Come to God about Everything that Concerns You
2. Pray and Supplicate with Thanksgiving
3. Think on These Things
4. Practice Daily

Step #1: Come to God about Everything that Concerns You
Our first instruction is mentioned immediately following the command for us not to worry. It's so simple that we sometimes miss it. It explains how we are to come to God in every circumstance and situation. It's says, "...**but in everything** by prayer and supplication, with thanksgiving, **let your requests be made known to God**" (NKJV emphasis added). Notice the parts in bold, "in everything... let your requests be known to God." We should make it a habit to come to God about any and everything that concerns us.

This means not just the big things. Don't wait until things get big to mention it to God if it's something that tempts us to worry. He loves us and wants to be involved in things we'd consider little, like not being able to find our car keys or being late for an appointment. Nothing is too small for God. If we ask the Holy Spirit to help us and He shows us where our keys are, it just confirms to us how important we are to Him and communicates to Him we are truly surrendering our lives to Him. Our trust in God and faith in Him increases.

Step #2: Pray and Supplicate with Thanksgiving

Next, Paul writes that by prayer, supplication (a petition), and thanksgiving the pressure of anxiety can be transcended by the peace of God. He says this is how we overcome worry and experience the peace of God operating in our lives.

> **Pray.** When we are talking to God about everything and in every situation no matter how big or small, God doesn't seem like a stranger to us. When we don't have a relationship with someone, we are uncomfortable talking to them.

For example, if someone has never talked to me and has never been to my house, when they come over, they might not feel comfortable asking me for a glass of water or going into my refrigerator even though they are thirsty. In the same manner, we do not want God to feel like a stranger to us. We need to establish a relationship with Him. The way to do that is to spend time with Him through His Word and prayer. Whenever we have a problem, a situation, or a challenge, and we are tempted to worry, we must pray.

What is Prayer?

- A personal conversation directed to God in casual, informal speech that acknowledges our total dependence on Him for resources and guidance for ourselves and others.
- Worship

The first definition is self-explanatory. However, I wanted to mention how the second definition relates in the context of our topic.

What is Worship?

Worship is the act—usually expressed in words or ceremony—of giving the highest esteem and reverent honor to God. Worship magnifies God. Worship doesn't magnify God because God is God, and we can't make God bigger. **What worship does is magnify God in our thinking.** As God is magnified in our thinking, our problem seems small because our perspective has changed.

Looking out the window of an airplane or from the top of a skyscraper, we notice how small things look. Worship changes our perspective. Suddenly, we are in God's presence, and then we look down on our problem from above. It doesn't seem as intimidating from above. God's Spirit instructs us in the truth that when we pause, get our mind off the problem, and worship Him, it will change our perspective.

In Philippians 4:11-13, the Apostle Paul further explains how praying about everything helps us to handle all of life's situations.

*...I have learned to be content [and self-sufficient through Christ, satisfied to the point where **I am not disturbed or uneasy] regardless of my circumstances**. I know how to get along and live humbly [in difficult times], and I also know how to enjoy abundance and live in prosperity. In any and every circumstance I have learned the secret [of facing life], whether well-fed or going hungry, whether having an abundance or being in need.*

I can do all things [which He has called me to do] through Him who strengthens and empowers me [to fulfill His purpose—I am self-sufficient in Christ's sufficiency; I am ready for anything and equal to anything through Him who infuses me with inner strength and confident peace.] (AMP emphasis added).

In other words, Paul is saying no matter where he finds himself, he has instructions on how to handle both pressure situations and prosperity. The reason he knows how to handle anything is because **he talks to God in all those situations.** Most Christians talk to God when they have pressure on them, but when they have prosperity, they don't pray. Believe it or not, it is just as challenging to stay free from worry when prospering as it is when we have a little. Paul said whether he's up or down, he prays and gives thanks in everything!

What does it mean to bring supplication to God?

In the Amplified Bible, it said, "by prayer and petition" and in the King James Version, it said, "by prayer and supplication" to make our requests known. A supplication is a petition that is a definite request. In other words, we are to come to God and **be specific** about what it is we desire. The more specific it is, the better. Once we've asked Him for specific assistance, we shouldn't turn around and try to fulfill the request ourselves! We need to learn to resist the temptation to do God's part. Whenever a challenge or problem comes up, **we** want to do something and solve it ourselves, but that's when we mess up. If what we've asked lines up with His promises, trust Him—who is the **source of peace and well-being**, according to Philippians 4:9 (AMP)—to handle it. Have faith in God.

"And the peace of God, which surpasses all understanding, will guard your hearts and minds through Christ Jesus" (Philippians 4:7 NKJV). The peace of God can't come from anyone else except Him.

What we need is peace not relief.

There is a difference between the peace of God and relief. The peace of God is an abiding spiritual force that will take us all the way through the situation. Relief is soulish and makes us feel better for a short period. For example, if we have a money problem and we want to do something, we go and borrow some money. We got relief through our own ingenuity, our own actions, and our own human efforts. However, that's only temporary because we borrowed it and will still have to find the money to pay it back and with interest!

When we go to people first before talking to God, we usually get human ideas, human opinions, and human thoughts, which brings us relief. God is sitting inside of us, questioning, "Why won't you talk to Me about this?"

When we follow His instructions and let our request be known to Him, Proverbs 16:3 says, "Commit your works to the LORD, and your thoughts will be established" (NKJV). The word *works* there means actions or activities. *Establish* means confirm, direct, order, frame, and settle. God says, "If you talk to Me about this challenge and commit your activities and actions to Me, I will confirm whether your thoughts are good or bad ideas. And if you're going the wrong way, I will set your thoughts in the right direction." I have learned this lesson the hard way.

Psalm 37:23 says, "The steps of a [good and righteous] man are directed and established by the LORD, and He delights in his way [and blesses his path]" (AMP). When I go to God and commit my works to Him, He will either confirm my thoughts, frame my thoughts, or set my thoughts right. Then when I began to walk in those thoughts, my steps are ordered. Then the Lord will delight in my way because my steps now came out of His thoughts.

Philippians 4:6-7 instructed us not to worry about anything, but in everything with prayer and supplication make our requests known to God. If we commit to Him, God promises to establish our thoughts, and then, the peace of God that surpasses all human understanding will guard our hearts and minds.

Make our request known with thanksgiving.

In Philippians 4:6, it said, "by prayer and petition **with thanksgiving**, continue to make your [specific] requests known to God" (AMP). The Living Bible gives further clarity, "Don't worry about anything; instead, pray about everything; tell God your needs, **and don't forget to thank him for his answers**" (emphasis added).

We should give thanks and praise to God in every circumstance, not because of the circumstance itself, but that God will reveal Himself as our problem solver, redeemer, and restorer of our peace.

When we talk to God first, we are not intimidated or in fear because we are looking at our problem from His perspective. He says after we make the definite request, thank Him for it.

When you've got a challenge, talk to God first, then make your request known with thanksgiving.

Step #3: Think on These Things

We can take control over worry and anxiety by replacing our thoughts with the listing in Philippians 4:8. We can't conquer worry if we're just thinking about everything that comes to our minds. When we find ourselves dwelling on the negative in a situation or envisioning destruction, think on these things.

Amplified Bible:
*"Finally, believers, whatever is true, whatever is honorable and worthy of respect, whatever is right and confirmed by God's word, whatever is pure and wholesome, whatever is lovely and brings peace, whatever is admirable and of good repute; if there is any excellence, if there is anything worthy of praise, **think continually on these things** [center your mind on them, and implant them in your heart]." (Emphasis added)*

King James Version:
"Finally, brethren, whatsoever things are true, whatsoever things are honest, whatsoever things are just, whatsoever things are pure, whatsoever things are lovely, whatsoever things are of good report; if there been a virtue, and if there be any praise, think on these things."

We should measure our thoughts by this list.

- If it is true, not false or imaginary, think on it.
- If it is honest, honorable, and worthy of respect, think on it.
- If it is just, right, impartial, and fair, think on that.
- If it is something holy, think on it.
- If it's lovely and promotes peace, think on it.
- If it is good news, think on it.
- If it is full of virtue, moral excellence, and integrity, think on it.
- If it is praiseworthy, commendable, worth talking about, think on it.

We're responsible for controlling our thoughts and we can always measure our feelings by our thoughts. If we get depressed, worried, anxious, or stressed, we are thinking about the wrong things.

Step #4: Practice Daily

*"The things which you have **learned** and received and heard **and seen in me**, **practice these things [in daily life]**, and the God [who is the source] of peace and well-being will be with you."* (Philippians 4:9 AMP emphasis added)

In these final instructions, Paul says to put into practice the things we've learned and to do it daily. Notice, he also mentioned "and seen in me." It's part of God's plan to teach us by example. So, we need to find a role model, someone who is already successful at where we're trying to go and observe how they are doing it. Then ask God for wisdom on our next steps.

One of the best testimonies we will ever have is how we handle and solve problems through the wisdom and power of Christ. If we can't handle problems, if we fall to pieces when it comes to problems and challenges, we're not going to be effective witnesses for Jesus Christ.

›› ASK YOURSELF...

Have I been coming to God about <u>everything</u> that concerns me?
Do I express worry or peace to those around me?
Am I praying and making <u>specific</u> requests to God?
Do others see me thanking God
even when I am experiencing trouble?
Is my life an effective witness for Jesus Christ?

›› APPLY WHAT YOU'VE LEARNED

Take the "Think on These Things" list from Philippians 4:8 and start to pay attention to what you are thinking. Throughout the day, when you have a thought that is the opposite of what is on the list, say out loud, "no, I am not going to think about that." And then purposely think about something else that is "lovely, of good report, brings peace, etc." Repeat daily.

CHAPTER 5

HANDLE THE IMPACT OF STRESS

*And there will be signs in the sun, in the moon, and in the stars; and on the earth **distress** of nations, with **perplexity**, the sea and the waves roaring; **men's hearts failing them from fear** and the expectation of those things which are coming on the earth, for the powers of the heavens will be shaken.* (Luke 21:25-26 NKJV emphasis added)

It says men's hearts are failing because they have gotten caught up in all the different things that are happening on the earth. We can get so caught up in all the things happening in our lives, our jobs, or school that it can shut down our hearts.

An improper response to stress can be hazardous to our mental and physical health and can lead to premature death.

One medical report reveals that 70 percent of all medical disorders are stress related. Chronic stress is often the contributing factor in many physical illnesses like headaches, muscle pain, and insomnia.

And it can cause high blood pressure, heart disease, elevated blood cholesterol levels, cancer, diabetes, digestive disorders, stomach pain, cramping, bloating, diarrhea, constipation, and ulcers.

Stress may also contribute to many mental disorders such as anger, anxiety attacks, depression, suicide, aggression, and abusive behavior. People get so stressed out they have mental or emotional breakdowns. They just shut down.

This isn't just my general observation. Read the following National Institute of Health (NIH) summary of stress-related physical and mental health illnesses and see *how very serious* stress is as an enemy to body, soul, and spirit:

> The relationship between stress and illness is complex. The susceptibility to stress varies from person to person. Among the factors that influenced the susceptibility to stress are genetic vulnerability, coping style, type of personality and social support. Not all stress has negative effect. Studies have shown that short-term stress boosted the immune system, but chronic stress has a significant effect on the immune system that ultimately manifest an illness. It raises catecholamine and suppressor T-cell levels, which suppress the immune system. This suppression, in turn raises the risk of viral infection. Stress also leads to the release of histamine, which can trigger severe broncho-constriction in asthmatics.

> Stress increases the risk for diabetes mellitus, especially in overweight individuals since psychological stress alters insulin needs. Stress also alters the acid concentration in the stomach, which can lead to peptic ulcers, stress ulcers or ulcerative colitis. Chronic stress can also lead to plaque buildup in the arteries (atherosclerosis), especially if combined with a high-fat diet and sedentary living. The correlation between stressful life events and psychiatric illness is stronger than the correlation with medical or physical illness.

The relationship of stress with psychiatric illness is strongest in neuroses, which is followed by depression and schizophrenia. There is no scientific evidence of a direct cause-and-effect relationship between the immune system changes and the development of cancer. However, recent studies found a link between stress, tumor development and suppression of natural killer (NK) cells, which is actively involved in preventing metastasis and destroying small metastases.[3]

What Is Stress?

1. A state of mental or emotional strain or pressure
2. Mental tension (perplexed)

*We are **pressured in every way** [hedged in], but not crushed; **perplexed** [unsure of finding a way out], but not driven to despair; **hunted down and persecuted, but not deserted** [to stand alone]; **struck down, but never destroyed;** always carrying around in the body the dying of Jesus, so that the [resurrection] life of Jesus also may be shown in our body. For we who live are constantly [experiencing the threat of] being handed over to death for Jesus' sake, so that the [resurrection] life of Jesus also may be evidenced in our mortal body [which is subject to death]. So physical death is [actively] at work in us, but [spiritual] life [is actively at work] in you. Yet we have the same spirit of faith as he had, who wrote in Scripture, "I* BELIEVED, THEREFORE I SPOKE*." We also believe, therefore we also speak, knowing that He who raised the Lord Jesus will also raise us with Jesus and will present us [along] with you in His presence. For all [these] things are for your sake, so that as [God's remarkable, undeserved] grace reaches to more and more people it may increase thanksgiving, to the glory of [our great] God.*

---

3 https://www.ncbi.nlm.nih.gov/pmc/articles/PMC3341916/

*Therefore **we do not become discouraged [spirit-less, disappointed, or afraid].** Though our outer self is [progressively] wasting away, yet our inner self is being [progressively] renewed day by day. For our momentary, light **distress [this passing trouble]** is producing for us an eternal weight of glory [a fullness] beyond all measure [surpassing all comparisons, a transcendent splendor and an endless blessedness]! So we look not at the things which are seen, but at the things which are unseen; for the things which are visible are temporal [just brief and fleeting], but the things which are invisible are everlasting and imper-ishable.* (2 Corinthians 4:8-18 AMP emphasis added)

The King James Version says Paul and his companions were "troubled on every side." They were pressured, perplexed, and persecuted. Trouble on every side means *hemmed in* on every side. Yet, he said they were "**not distressed**." This means they were **not stressed** about it because they didn't allow their stressful circumstances to pilfer their thoughts or emotions. They were "perplexed, but were not in despair." He said we were hunted down and persecuted, but we did not feel forsaken or abandoned or deserted. We were struck down but not destroyed.

To be perplexed means to be at a loss mentally (not knowing what to do or how to handle the negative stress). In other words, Paul was saying...

**Refuse to be distressed by stress,
disturbed by disturbances,
or grieved by grievances!**

We should reject rejection and stay encouraged instead of discouraged. Paul continues to explain why they were not in despair, not feeling dejected, and not discouraged. It was because they had an amazing "treasure in earthen vessels, that the excellency of the **power may be of God, and not of us**" (2 Corinthians 4:7 KJV emphasis added). We don't let problems overwhelm us because of the One who lives on the inside of us.

In Philippians 4:11-13, Paul writes he learned to be content no matter what the outside circumstances might be. He knew he could "do all things through Christ" who strengthened him (NKJV). The Amplified Bible says, "I can do all things [which He has called me to do] through Him who strengthens *and* empowers me [to fulfill His purpose—I am self-sufficient in Christ's sufficiency; I am ready for anything and equal to anything through Him who infuses me with inner strength and confident peace.]" The J. B. Phillips translation reads, "I am ready for anything through the strength of the one who lives within me."

Declare and Confess:

- *In Christ, I have the power not to be discouraged, spiritless, disappointed, afraid, or distressed.*
- *In Christ, I have the strength and ability to overcome.*
- *I am empowered to win no matter what enemy attacks me.*

Replace Inner Chaos with Enduring Peace

In 2 Corinthians 1, the Apostle Paul is writing to the church at Corinth. He begins by praying for them to experience inner calm and spiritual well-being from the God of all comfort and encouragement. In turn, they could comfort and encourage others in distress with the same level of comfort they had received from God themselves.

> *Grace to you and **peace [inner calm and spiritual well-being] from God** our Father and the Lord Jesus Christ. Blessed [gratefully praised and adored] be the God and Father of our Lord Jesus Christ, the Father of mercies and the **God of all comfort, who comforts and encourages us in every trouble so that we will be able to***

comfort and encourage those who are in any kind of trouble, with the comfort with which we ourselves are comforted by God. For just as Christ's sufferings are ours in abundance [as they overflow to His followers], so also our comfort [our reassurance, our encouragement, our consolation] is abundant through Christ [it is truly more than enough to endure what we must]. But if we are troubled and distressed, it is for your comfort and salvation; or if we are comforted and encouraged, it is for your comfort, which works [in you] when you patiently endure the same sufferings which we experience. And our hope for you [our confident expectation of good for you] is firmly grounded [assured and unshaken], since we know that just as you share as partners in our sufferings, so also you share as partners in our comfort. For we do not want you to be uninformed, brothers and sisters, about our trouble... (2 Corinthians 1:2-8a AMP emphasis added)

Being in Christ makes a difference. When issues arise, we don't have to fall apart. We can have peace and comfort. Ask God for His peace that surpasses all understanding and His comfort.

Our Heavenly Father is the God of all comfort who comforts us when there's tension, strain, and pressure in our lives.

We know and are confident that regardless of what's happening around us, God will help us no matter what we are facing. This includes all kinds of pressures. Sometimes, there's pressure applied to our flesh to sin. That's what temptation is. Sometimes, our pressure comes against our minds. Sometimes, we have family pressure, relationship pressure, or marital pressure. Other times, it is the pressure of dealing with our children. Sometimes, it's a job or financial pressure. The

Bible declares He's the God of **all** comfort, no matter what we face.

**God comforts us so we can help others
who are experiencing pressure, strain,
and tension in their lives.**

Verse 4 exhorts, "[God] who comforts and encourages us in every trouble so that we will be able to comfort and encourage those who are in any kind of trouble, with the comfort with which we ourselves are comforted by God." This reminds me of a testimony a Christian man shared with me. He said God gave him peace and comfort when his Christian grandmother passed away. Because of it, he was able to read a poem filled with hope and faith at this grandmother's funeral which brought comfort to other members of the family. That's the way it's supposed to be. Christians should encourage and comfort one another with the comfort the Spirit gives us.

Paul goes on to explain, "For just as Christ's sufferings are ours in abundance [as they overflow to His followers], so also our comfort [our reassurance, our encouragement, our consolation] is abundant through Christ [it is truly more than enough to endure what we must]. But if we are troubled and distressed, it is for your comfort and salvation; or if we are comforted and encouraged, it is for your comfort, which works [in you] when you patiently endure the same sufferings which we experience. And our hope for you [our confident expectation of good for you] is firmly grounded [assured and unshaken], since we know that just as you share as partners in our sufferings, so also you share as partners in our comfort."

Some stress we experience is not because we have done anything wrong. Some of the things we experience are because we are doing things right. Christ didn't suffer because He did something wrong. He suffered because He was doing something right.

Don't internalize the suffering and the pressure. Instead, receive the comfort God has for you.

Paul continues, "For we would not brethren, have you ignorant of our trouble." *Trouble* means pressure. Paul was experiencing pressure.

Indeed, we felt within ourselves that we had received the sentence of death [and were convinced that we would die, but this happened] so that we would not trust in ourselves, but in God who raises the dead. **He rescued us** *from so great a threat of death,* **and will continue to rescue us. On Him we have set our hope.** *And He will again rescue us [from danger and draw us near], while you join in helping us by your prayers. Then thanks will be given by many persons on our behalf for the gracious gift [of deliverance] granted to us through the prayers of many [believers].* (2 Corinthians 1:9-11 AMP emphasis added)

The pressure they were dealing with was beyond their natural ability and human strength to handle. They needed more than human strength. In fact, they were at the point they thought they were going to die because they could not figure out how they were going to get out of it. Paul is teaching us when we get to the point of when we don't know how to handle the tension, strain, and pressure, we need to trust in God. **When they trusted God, He delivered them.** They remembered what God had done in the past and that produced confidence and hope for the present and the future.

Paul knew that if we are on this earth, we will experience trouble and pressure. However, he knew the way to handle all his overwhelming trouble. "And He will again rescue us [from danger and draw us near], while you join in helping us by your prayers. Then thanks will be given by many persons on our behalf for the gracious gift [of deliverance] granted to us through the prayers of many [believers]."

Paul expressed two things. He knew God would come to their rescue and he knew others were praying for them.

Prayer Overcomes Stress

There is a seedtime harvest principle in prayer. When we pray for somebody else, we sow a seed into their lives. We may not know what they are going through, but our prayers can help them through the pressure they might be facing. If God puts someone on our heart to pray for, please stop everything and pray for them right then.

Sometimes, when we are experiencing pressure, we don't want to go to church, read the Bible, or pray. When we have pressure, that's exactly when we need to pray!

Stress is tension, mental tension, strain, and pressure. Stress is a way of life in the sense we all face external pressure. However, the good news of the gospel is we don't have to be victimized by external pressure. We don't have to allow the pressure to get inside of us.

**As we pray without ceasing,
we can have pressure all around us
and have peace on the inside.**

In John 17:15-17, Jesus is praying knowing He was soon returning to heaven. "I pray not that thou shouldest take them out of the world, but that thou shouldest keep them from the evil. They are not of the world, even as I am not of the world. Sanctify them through thy truth: thy word is truth" (KJV).

In other words, Jesus knew His disciples were going to experience pressure while they were still on this earth. He knew they had a mission before them to go into all the world and share the truth they had learned from Him. He had taught them that if they would pray and seek God, He would set them apart and protect them from the evil that would try to prevent them from handling the pressure.

What Can Cause Stress?

Let's identify a few causes of stress and then I will reveal practical tips for reducing the stress in your life.

Causes:

1. Positive events can cause stress.
   a. A wedding. It can be extremely stressful to the point of impacting the night of the honeymoon.
   b. The birth of a baby. I remember when my son, Michael K., was born. I had pressure on me because this newborn depended on me. I had to take care of him.
   c. Retirement, a new job, or a promotion.
   d. A new home.
   e. Vacation planning.
2. The inability to adapt to our surroundings (e.g., work, home, church).
3. Competitive pursuit of wealth and prestige can overwhelm and consume a person over time. (e.g., extra jobs)
4. Poverty and scarcity.
5. Overwhelming demands and responsibilities can cause feelings we have too much to do and not enough time or resources to get it all done.
6. Fear of failure or failure to achieve a goal.
7. Unexpected major events such as a serious illness, an accident, the death of a loved one, the loss of a job, and divorce are big stressors.
8. Minor events (e.g., missing car keys/cell phone, a flat tire, locking the keys in the car/house, forgetting an appointment, lost papers, traffic jams, having company over for dinner).
9. Academic pressure such as grades, upcoming tests, and homework.

Practical Tips to Reduce Stress in Your Life

Here are ten simple, yet practical things, that will help us overcome stress. Use this list to evaluate and adjust as needed to move toward a stress-free life.

1. **Do one thing at a time until the project is completed**, then go on to something else. It's wonderful if we have the capacity to multitask and juggle several projects. However, if we find ourselves becoming tense and stressed, then we must take a step back and decide to focus on one task at a time until we finish it.

   In my past, I felt like I needed a "harvest" in every area of my life. I wanted to see fruit achieved in my marriage, my children, my job, and my church. I discovered that attacking one area at a time and achieving victory in one at a time was better for my mental health. In the long run, it made me more productive.

2. **Get organized.** Make a to-do list. Let's say you have an appointment tomorrow. You should get organized and plan for the appointment tonight. Do not leave everything until tomorrow morning; that causes unnecessary stress. Choose the clothes you want to wear tonight. Check your car tonight and see if you have enough gas. Check your navigation app to see how long it'll take to drive there. Set the alarm clock with the amount of time you need to shower, eat breakfast, and get there early.

3. **Know your pressure capacity/bandwidth and delegate.** Sometimes, we're tense and stressed because we are doing things somebody else could be doing (e.g., have the kids do household chores, pay for someone to mow the lawn, fully delegate tasks to your employees).

4. **Stop procrastinating.** *Procrastination* is putting off doing something. For instance, every time you go into the garage or closet, you keep saying you will clean it, and you do not. It causes you stress. Every time you delay having a tough conversation with someone, you add to your stress level. Whatever it is that you have

been avoiding, go ahead and do it.

5. **Laugh often**. One of my favorite Scriptures in the Bible is Proverbs 17:22 which says, "A merry heart, does good, like medicine, but a broken spirit dries the bones" (NKJV). Laughter is a wonderful thing that can release some of life's pressures. The New Living Translation says, "A cheerful heart is good medicine, but a broken spirit saps a person's strength."

   Years ago, my father was ill, so I quit my job and came home to help my mother with my dad's care. Caregivers experience a lot of stress, and I was exhausted. Dad deteriorated mentally and physically. He deteriorated to the point where he couldn't feed himself. The doctors finally told us there was nothing more they could do for him. Suddenly, the Spirit of God came on me. I started laughing while I was driving in my car, and I just could not stop. Right in the middle of that trouble, God gave me laughter. Find something to laugh about and you will be amazed at what it does for you. It truly is like a medicine.

6. **Engage in regular exercise. Keep physically fit.** 1 Timothy 4:8 says it is important to engage in both physical and spiritual training. Healthcare professionals recommend regular exercise to relieve stress. Get your body moving!

7. **Honor the Sabbath principle.** In Mark 2:27, Jesus said to them, "The Sabbath was made for man, not man for the Sabbath" (AMP). God instituted a work/rest cycle. Six days you work, one day you rest. When you work all the time, you are violating the Sabbath principle and you're opening yourself up to sickness, stress, and all kinds of things. Take a day off!

8. **Take a vacation**. Mark 6:31 reads, "He said to them, 'Come away by yourselves to a secluded place and rest a

little while'—for there were many [people who were continually] coming and going, and they could not even find time to eat" (AMP). If you can't go to the Bahamas, you can certainly go to a city an hour away from your home. Vacate!

9. **Take a nap. Stay rested.** You will be absolutely amazed at how a nap will make a difference in your stress level. In fact, in some countries, employers have a scheduled nap time built into the day. The companies shut down and the employees take a nap because they have discovered people can produce more after taking a nap. Reduce stress by incorporating a 15-, 20-, or 30-minute nap into your schedule. The results will be great for your mental and physical health.

10. **Spend time meditating in God's Word**. Use your breath to breathe in part of a verse and breathe out the second part. Silence all the random chatter in your mind. Be still and know God. Listen to the still, small voice of His Spirit. Focus on the truth of God's Word not the myths of the world that seek to distract you. Stay focused on what pleases God not what pleases man.

›› ASK YOURSELF…

Have I gotten so caught up in all the things happening in my life that it has caused mental health issues or a constant feeling of stress?

When I am experiencing pressure in my life, do I stop going to church, reading the Bible, and praying?

›› APPLY WHAT YOU'VE LEARNED

Review the 10 practical tips to reduce stress. For each tip, ask yourself, "What adjustments can I make in this area?" Gradually implement changes one at time.

CHAPTER 6

SET THE RIGHT PRIORITIES FOR STRESS-FREE LIVING

*Come to Me, all you who labor and are heavy-laden and over-burdened, and **I will cause you to rest. [I will ease and relieve and refresh your souls.]***
*Take My yoke upon you and learn of Me, for I am gentle (meek) and humble (lowly) in heart, and **you will find rest (relief and ease and refreshment and recreation and blessed quiet) for your souls.** For My yoke is wholesome (useful, good—not harsh, hard, sharp, or pressing, but comfortable, gracious, and pleasant), and My burden is **light and easy** to be borne.* (Matthew 11:28-30 AMPC emphasis added)

Jesus said He would ease and relieve and refresh our souls. Our soul is made up of our mind, will, and emotions. This means it is possible to live without feeling stressed. Here are four keys to a stress-free life.

1. Perception (How we see things)
2. Personal Responsibility
3. Priorities
4. Persevering, Persistent Trust

Key #1: Perception

The Egyptians pursued them, all the horses and chariots of Pharaoh and his horsemen and his army, and overtook them encamped at the [Red] Sea by Pi-hahiroth, in front of Baal-zephon. When Pharaoh drew near, the Israelites looked up, and behold, the Egyptians were marching after them; and the **Israelites were exceedingly frightened and cried out to the Lord***.*

And they said to Moses, Is it because there are no graves in Egypt that you have taken us away to die in the wilderness? Why have you treated us this way and brought us out of Egypt? Did we not tell you in Egypt, Let us alone; let us serve the Egyptians? For it would have been better for us to serve the Egyptians than to die in the wilderness. **Moses told the people, Fear not; stand still (firm, confident, undismayed) and see the salvation of the Lord which He will work for you today.** *For the Egyptians you have seen today you shall never see again.* (Exodus 14:9-13 AMPC emphasis added)

In Exodus 14, God brought Israel out of Egyptian bondage. They had been in bondage for over 430 years, and they were now encamped at the Red Sea. Pharaoh changed his mind and decided he was going to recapture them. This sounds like a pressure-filled situation, right? Notice the two perceptions of what was happening: **Fear vs. Faith.** The Israelites were exceedingly frightened, but Moses told the people, "Fear not; stand still (firm, confident, undismayed) and see the salvation of the Lord which He will work for you today."

Perception is how we see a situation, a thing, or a person. Perception is our mental response or mindset.

The Israelites looked at their situation and they saw failure, defeat, bondage, failure, and destruction. They saw the horses and the chariots, and said, "We should have stayed in Egyptian bondage; we were better off in Egypt." On the other hand, Moses looked at the same situation and saw success, deliverance, and salvation. His exhortation was, "Fear not, stand still and see the salvation of the Lord." It was the same situation, yet polar opposite perceptions.

Perception is determined by our focus.

The Israelites focused on the problem, while Moses saw the possibility and potential for God's miraculous intervention. Whenever we focus on the problem, we will end up with a negative perception. Moses focused on the answer.

Whenever we focus on the answer, we will always end up with a positive perception.

In fact, in Hebrews 11:27, it says, "It was by faith that Moses left the land of Egypt, not fearing the king's anger. He kept right on going because he kept his eyes on the one who is invisible" (NLT).

Perception can either ease or intensify stress.

Whenever we are focused on the problem, the stress in our life will be intensified. Whenever our focus is on the answer it will ease the stress. We want the stress to be eased. To achieve this, there are several things we must do.

1. We must control our thought life.

The battle is always in the mind. 2 Corinthians 10:3-5 says we don't war after the flesh. We are in a spiritual battle against our spiritual enemy. As we learned in a previous chapter, we are going to have to control our thought life in order to battle the lies of this enemy. The enemy will try to get us to listen to negative thoughts like...

It's all over.
You might as well just quit and give up.
You should just kill yourself.
You're not going to win.
You're not going to make it.
You'll never get it.

The truth is nobody can control our thought life, but us. When we have fearful thoughts in anticipation of something bad happening, our perception is off focus. We have control. Cast down that imagination.

2. We must not focus on the problem.
When we focus on the problem, we magnify the problem. A classic illustration of that is found in 1 Samuel 17. The Philistines were at war with Israel, and they had a giant called Goliath. He was nearly 10 feet tall, weighed approximately 400 pounds, had armor that weighed 125 pounds, a spear that had an iron tip that weighed 15 pounds. He was a formidable opponent. He would stand in the valley and say to the armies of the living God "...give me a man so that we may fight together. When King Saul and all Israel heard these words of the Philistine, **they were dismayed and greatly afraid**" (Verse 10b-11 AMP). He was relentless. He appeared every morning and evening for 40 days with taunts and threats. As every Israelite looked at, listened to, and focused on the problem day after day, the problem became bigger and bigger in their minds.

David, a youth with no military experience, was on the backside of the desert, worshiping the Lord, meditating on God's Word, and tending to his father's sheep. He came on the scene and heard Goliath and was shocked at what he was saying and Israel's fearful reaction. He hadn't been looking at the problem, listening to the problem, or focusing on the problem for 40 days and 40 nights. He had been listening to God.

David said the same Lord that delivered him from the lion and the bear would help him to be victorious against the giant. He told Goliath in verse 45, "You come to me with a sword, a spear, and a javelin, but I come to you in the name of the LORD of hosts, the God of the armies of Israel, whom you have taunted" (AMP). Oftentimes, we sit at night meditating and thinking about the issue. Next, the problem will begin to speak to us and keep our focus on it rather than on God. Then we start saying (confessing) the negative, fearful outcomes that have consumed us. We must **not** focus on the problem.

3. Stop focusing on the smaller, negative aspects of the situation. Focus on the greater positive aspects and possibilities of the situation. Stay focused. Reject every distraction. In every situation, there are going to be negatives. However, if we would think about the whole scenario of our lives, we will find more positives than negatives. The challenge is we end up focusing on the negative and neglect the positive. I call that the Eve Syndrome.

And the LORD God commanded the man, saying, "You may freely (unconditionally) eat [the fruit] from every tree of the garden; but [only] from the tree of the knowledge (recognition) of good and evil you shall not eat, otherwise on the day that you eat from it, you shall most certainly die [because of your disobedience]. (Genesis 2:16-17 AMP)

Because the enemy deceived Eve, she began to concentrate on the **one** tree they couldn't eat. There was a garden filled with other fruit-bearing trees available to them. Satan diverted her attention from all the positive benefits and blessings she had and centered her attention on what she did not have, which was a tactic from the enemy if we allow it. When we find ourselves focusing on the **one** bad part of the good situation, arrest the thought immediately and replace it with the positives.

It is like the parent whose child has two A's, two B's, and a C on their report card. The parent immediately says, "I noticed you got a

C." The emphasis was on a perceived failure versus the positivity of the A's and B's. What matters most is not the problem or situation but how we see it and respond to it.

Key #2: Personal Responsibility

And the Lord said to Moses, "Why do you cry to Me? Tell the children of Israel to go forward... Then Moses stretched out his hand over the sea; and the Lord caused the sea to go back by a strong east wind all that night, and made the sea into dry land, and the waters were divided." (Exodus 14:15, 21 NKJV)

Four Principles Concerning Personal Responsibility

1. We are responsible for doing the possible, and then trust God to do the impossible. Moses stretched forth his hand. That's possible. The Lord caused the sea to recede. That's the impossible. In every situation, we must ask ourselves, "What is it that I can possibly do?" Why? Because we are responsible for *our* part. God never moves supernaturally until people first do what they are capable of doing. Oftentimes, we are waiting for God to move. God did not perform the miracle of dividing the sea until Moses did what he was supposed to do. In this case, Moses' part was to obey the Word of the Lord.

In 2 Kings 4:1-7, there was a widow woman whose husband had died. The creditors were on their way to take her sons in lieu of the debt her husband owed. She cried out to the prophet Elisha, who asked her, "What do you have in your house?"

...She said, "Your maidservant has nothing in the house except a [small] jar of [olive] oil." Then he said, "Go, borrow containers from all your neighbors, empty containers— and not just a few. Then you shall go in and shut the door behind you and your sons, and pour out [the oil you have] into all these containers, and you shall set aside each one

when it is full. (Verses 2-4 AMP)

Everything at this point was within her power to do. Nothing supernatural had happened yet. However, she did her part.

So she left him and shut the door behind her and her sons; they were bringing her the containers as she poured [the oil]. ⁶ When the containers were all full, she said to her son, "Bring me another container." And he said to her, "There is not a one left." Then the oil stopped [multiplying]. ⁷ Then she came and told the man of God. He said, "Go, sell the oil and pay your debt, and you and your sons can live on the rest. (Verses 5-7 AMP)

Notice, once she did her part, that's when the supernatural took place. That little pot of oil just kept pouring! God multiplied what she had. If she had done a little bit more by getting more containers, God would have continued multiplying it. The oil didn't flow until **after** she did what she was capable of doing. This is a lesson for all of us.

God rarely creates something from scratch or produces something that does not require the active participation of the recipients. A classic illustration of that is in Matthew 14:13-20 and the feeding of the 5,000 men plus women and children.

"When it was evening, His disciples came to Him, saying, "This is a deserted place, and the hour is already late. Send the multitudes away, that they may go into the villages and buy themselves food." (Verse 15 NKJV)

Jesus already knew what He was going to do.

"But Jesus said to them, 'They do not need to go away. You give them something to eat.' And they said to Him, 'We have here only five loaves and two fish.' He said, 'Bring them here to Me.' Then He commanded the multitudes to sit down on

the grass. And He took the five loaves and the two fish, and looking up to heaven, He blessed and broke and gave the loaves to the disciples; and the disciples gave to the multitudes. So they all ate and were filled, and they took up twelve baskets full of the fragments that remained." (Verses 16-20 NKJV)

Everyone had a role in the miracle. The disciples had to do their part and the people had to follow instructions to receive. **Then,** the supernatural happened! God takes what we have, whether it is our finances, our talent, our time, or our ability and He requires our active participation.

God does not operate solo.
He invites us to partner with Him.
He desires that we participate with Him.
When we do our part,
God does the impossible!

---

2. Do not stress out about things outside of our control. For example, in Exodus, Moses told Pharaoh that God said, "Let My people go." Pharaoh's response was beyond Moses' control, and thus was not part of his responsibility. God wanted the people to follow Moses, but Moses could not make the people follow him. That was outside of his control. Could Moses split the Red Sea? No, that was exceedingly beyond his control.

Stressing out about things we can't control,
can't change, and have no responsibility for, is
not good for our mental health. Although this
takes practice, decide not to be concerned.

---

3. Realize, not every need is our responsibility. Some things are within our power, but they are not our responsibility. We could do something about it, but we need to make sure we're not carrying someone else's load. We could feed the neighbor's children, but is it our responsibility? No. It is not our duty to meet every need that arises. For instance, we may know someone struggling to pay their bills. They mention to us that they are being evicted from their apartment this week. I'm not saying we should never help others. **I'm saying don't make other people's responsibilities our own.** This can lead to undue stress.

4. Find out our responsibility in every situation, do our part, and rest. We can avoid a lot of stress if we stop and take the time to evaluate our personal responsibility. I used to worry about everything. As a pastor, I saw every problem, every situation, and people having hard times. I was stressed out. Then, the Lord told me my responsibility was to be an example to the flock, feed the flock, study, pray, and receive the Word from Heaven to provide spiritual food that will make a difference in the flock's everyday life. He told me I was to provide the leadership and train the leadership base so they could minister as well. I was to encourage the members to love each other, minister to each of them, and then I was supposed to rest in it. However, I was stressed about church growth (or the lack thereof at the time). God spoke to me and told me to "do your part, rest, and the church will grow." God's part was the church growth. Resting in what He told me was my responsibility.

Key #3: Priorities

> *"For God is not the author of confusion, but of peace...,*
> (1 Corinthians 14:33a KJV)

The Bible says God is not the author of confusion. He is a God of *order*. Verse 40 says, "Let all things be done decently and in order" (KJV). That means in sequence, according to an arrangement, or according to rank. In other words, there's order in the universe and there should be order in our lives. To achieve order, we need to decide what our priorities are in life.

Our priority as a believer is our relationship with the Lord and then everything else should trinkle down from there.

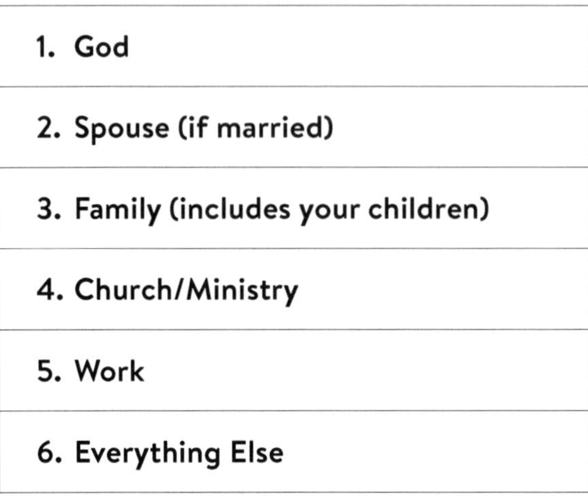

When our priorities are right, it will ease stress.

Let's read the story of Jesus' visit to the home of Martha and Mary. Each sister had to choose their priority. Martha chose to serve. Mary chose to sit at Jesus' feet.

Which sister was stressed out?
Which one was at peace?
Which one do you want to be?

Now while they were on their way, Jesus entered a village [called Bethany], and a woman named Martha welcomed Him into her home. She had a sister named Mary, who seated herself at the Lord's feet and was continually listening to His *teaching. But **Martha was very busy and distracted with all of her serving responsibilities;** and she approached Him and said, "Lord, is it of no concern to You that my sister has left me to do the serving alone? Tell her to help me and do her part." But the Lord replied to her, **"Martha, Martha, you are worried and bothered and anxious about so many things; but only one thing is necessary, for Mary has chosen the good part** [that which is to her advantage], which will not be taken away from her."* (Luke 10:38-42 AMP emphasis added)

Learn How to Set Right Priorities

1. Recognize that some things are urgent, while others are important. Urgent things call for immediate attention. Jesus told Martha she was stressed and troubled about many urgent things. She was stressed and troubled about the cooking, the serving, and the cleaning. On the other hand, some things are important. Important things are weighty matters, issues of superior worth, and value. Important things are things that must be given priority. In this scenario, listening to the words of Jesus was an important thing. Martha chose the urgent things. Mary chose the important thing.

Our personal devotional time should be an important priority. Some Christians are zealous in their church attendance, but lax in their personal, private relationship with the Lord. Spiritual growth, development, and real success will come from the quiet time we spend with God, studying His Word, fellowshipping with Him, and praying. This has sustained my life since I was saved in 1977. I get up early and spend the first hour of my day doing this. **Many times, our problem is we allow urgent things to take us away from the important things.** If we don't pray and spend time with the Lord and feed our spirit, then we are feeding our flesh. Whatever we feed is going to control our lives. The more out of control our flesh becomes, the more stress we'll experience.

2. It is the wise person who balances the urgent and the important. In Mark 1:16-20, Jesus saw Simon and Andrew casting a net into the sea because they were fisherman. "Jesus said unto them, 'Come ye after me and I will make you to become fishers of men.' And straightway, they forsook their nets, and followed him. And when he had gone a little farther thence, he saw James the son of Zebedee, and John his brother who also were in the ship, mending their nets. And straightway he called them: and they left their father Zebedee in the ship with the hired servants, and went after him" (KJV).

Calling a group of men who would be an extension of His ministry was important because Jesus knew He was going to only be here on earth for three-and-a-half years. He had to have a group of men who would carry this gospel into the earth. He was tending to important matters.

Shortly after, we see Jesus going into the synagogue to teach. While there, a man with an unclean spirit interrupted Him. Jesus rebuked him. Jesus was balancing the urgent with the important. He called those men. That was important. He taught in the synagogue. That was important. Then, He dealt with that urgent matter (unclean spirit), but He never allowed the urgent to take Him away from the important.

Verses 29-31 reads, "and forthwith, when they were come out of the synagogue, they entered into the house of Simon and Andrew, with James and John. But Simon's wife's mother lay sick of a fever..." There's another urgent situation. "And he came and took her by the hand, and lifted her up; And immediately the fever left her, and she ministered unto them" (KJV).

Jesus continues to minister and heal for the rest of the day. Then, verse 35 says, "And in the morning, rising up a great while before day, he went out and departed into a solitary place, and there prayed." You'd think He'd be sleeping in, wouldn't you? No, **He had to tend to the important before the urgent showed up.**

Jesus kept the important where it should be. It is the wise person who knows how to balance the urgent and the important. If we get caught up in needs all the time, we'll never have time to do the important. There will always be needs such as cleaning the house, paying bills, and doing laundry. There are endless needs. Therefore, learn to balance the urgent and the important.

3. There will be times when you must say "no" to the urgent in order to do the important. Don't go on a guilt trip when that happens. Mark 1:36-38 says after Jesus left early to go pray, "...Simon and those who were with Him searched for Him. When they found Him, they said to Him, 'Everyone is looking for You.' But He said to them, 'Let us go into the next towns, that I may preach there also, because for this purpose I have come forth'" (NKJV). Peter tells Him everyone is looking for Him and expects Him to go back to those needs, but Jesus says, there are some other places He needs to go.

There will be times when we must say *no* to the urgent in order to do the important.

If we don't learn how to say no, we'll always
be stressed out because we're doing things we
aren't supposed to do right now.

---

4. You cannot fulfill everybody's expectations and live a priority-focused life.

"Now a certain man was sick, named Lazarus, of Bethany, the town of Mary and her sister Martha. (It was that Mary which anointed the Lord with ointment, and wiped his feet with her hair, whose brother Lazarus was sick.) Therefore his sisters sent unto him, saying, Lord, behold, he whom thou lovest is sick. When Jesus heard that, he said, This sickness is not unto death, but for the glory of God, that the Son of God might be glorified thereby. Now Jesus loved Martha, and her sister, and Lazarus. When he had heard therefore that he was sick, he abode two days still in the same place where he was." (John 11:1-6 KJV)

They all expected Jesus to drop everything He was doing because the one He loved was sick, but He stayed right where He was for two more days. "And many of the Jews came to Martha and Mary, to comfort them concerning their brother. [He died.] Then Martha, as soon as she heard that Jesus was coming, went and met him: And Mary sat still in the house. Then Martha said unto Jesus, Lord if thou hadst been here, my brother had not died" (verses 19-21, 32 KJV emphasis added). Both Martha and Mary were frustrated and disappointed because things did not happen as they expected.

The challenge when we live a priority-focused life is there are going to be some people who are going to be angry, mad, frustrated, and disappointed when we do not meet their expectations.

Never let circumstances or people distract you from the godly priorities of your life. You won't be able to meet everyone's expectations. Attempting to do so will result in the opposite of a stress-free life.

Key #4: Persevering, Persistent Trust

When the Bible says to *trust* in the Lord, it doesn't mean being passive. It means we must actively determine our role, our responsibility, and our obligation. Then, we trust God to do His part. We get stressed out and frustrated because we're trying to do God's part. **Don't try to do God's part.** Trust Him.

›› ASK YOURSELF...

Do I know what my part is?
Am I trying to do God's part?
Am I allowing urgent needs to distract me from the important?

›› PRAYER DURING TIMES OF STRESS

Heavenly Father,

You know what's going on with me right now. I am casting my care on You because I know You care for me. Although I'm in the middle of a stressful situation, I am experiencing Your tangible peace which surpasses all understanding and a calmness in the storm. I am anxious for nothing. I am not concerned about things outside of my control. Reveal any areas of my life that I need to reprioritize or where I need to adjust my perception. I want to focus on what is the most important. Thank You, Father God, for always being a present help in my time of need.

In Jesus' name, Amen.

CHAPTER 7

REALIZE DISCOURAGEMENT IS AN ENEMY

Hope deferred makes the heart sick. But when the desire comes, it is a tree of life. (Proverbs 13:12 NKJV)

I know something about discouragement. I have been saved since October 4, 1977. I have been pastoring for over 40 years. We all have our challenges in some form or fashion. Out of all the things people deal with, I think the area I have struggled with the most has been this area of discouragement. In fact, it took me years to realize I was truly battling with an enemy I had allowed to infiltrate my life. I thought it was just a feeling or an emotion in response to the challenges in my life. It took me years to get a handle on and learn how to battle this enemy of my peace called discouragement.

I found that anytime or anywhere satan has enjoyed any successes in our life, whether it is with lust, stealing, greed, anger, or whatever, we need to understand that even after we win and we drive him out, we must be ready for him to come back.

Throughout my life, I have learned to drive out discouragement. I know what it is, and I know how to handle it. I have also learned what to do when it tries to come back. I know it will often rise up and show its ugly head. I can leave church some Sundays, have a church full of folks, rejoice over the people who have gotten saved, and then on Sunday night, discouragement shows up at the door of my thinking. I'd like to share with you what I've learned about how to drive out this enemy of discouragement, so it does not try to steal, kill, or destroy your hope.

Hope reveals our dream, shows us our goal, and gives us our vision.

We should all have a vision on an individual level and then on a corporate level. All of us need vision for ourselves individually, our family and our marriage (if we're married). We should have a vision for a better life. We should have a vision for...

- our career
- our education
- our business
- our happiness

All of us have some form of vision, something we are shooting for, and some goal to reach. Proverbs 29:18a reads, "Where there is no vision, the people perish..." (KJV). We must have a vision in life to be prosperous and successful.

One of the most powerful and destructive enemies that will come against our vision is discouragement. I have learned that true visions from God are things that really matter in life and aren't achieved overnight. It is true we live in a fast-paced, get-rich-quick, and immediate gratification society. We've got the express lanes and kiosks at banks and grocery stores. Our society is filled with microwaves and air fryers to cook food in minutes instead of hours, curbside pickup, and overnight delivery on almost anything we can order online. When we post on social media, we expect to receive immediate feedback through likes and loves. We have a mindset that says everything must be quick, or we become impatient and even discouraged.

However, in the kingdom of God, a divine law of growth, process, and progress is in place. For the most part, in the natural world, people are **not** successful overnight, even if it appears as such on social media. Therefore, we must be willing to hold onto our vision and our dream and allow God to guide us through our journey to His goal for our lives. That also means we are going to have to learn how to overcome discouragement when things do not occur as quickly and in the way we think they should.

To do this successfully, we need to understand what this enemy discouragement looks like and acts like by describing and defining it. To defeat this enemy, we need to be able to recognize him and the weapons he tries to use against us.

#1: Discouraged means *to be deprived of or lacking courage.* Courage is the attitude needed to face and deal with anything recognized as dangerous, difficult, or painful. Instead of withdrawing from it, we deal with it. We don't run from the issues, problems, or challenges before us. We face them. Therefore, if the word *discouraged* means to be deprived of courage, it means we are deprived of the ability to face and deal with danger, difficulty, pain, or trouble.

To be discouraged also means *to be disheartened which causes us to lose hope or confidence.* It also means *to become dispirited, a lowering of our spirits* which can cause us to have a loss of drive, a loss of enthusiasm, and a loss of energy. At that point, we become fatigued, weary, and just plain tired.

In fact, one of the strategies of the enemy is to bombard our minds with so much confusion, negativity, and impatience that we are worn down, fatigued, and weary of well-doing. The evil one wants us to get so fatigued and discouraged that we cannot function.

 # 2: Discouraged means *to be dissuaded, neutralized, and to stop our activity.*
We choose to be neutral instead of proactive, impatient instead of patient, complaining instead of thanking, and negative instead of positive. In fact, we choose to trust the god of this world who says

impossible, instead of trusting the Omnipotent God who declares that *all things are possible* (Mark 10:27).

Whatever we are doing that's good, whether it be getting in the Word, meditating on the Word, praying, witnessing, giving, or loving, satan wants to dissuade us and stop us from doing it.

#3: Discouraged means *to impede forward movement.*

We may be doing well and going forward toward achieving our goals, but then, suddenly, discouragement comes in to impede our forward movement.

The kingdom of this world belongs to satan. It's a cancel culture attacking the Kingdom of God. The enemy of our soul seeks to cancel courage with discouragement, peace with warfare, love with hate, confidence with second guessing, and faith with doubt.

Satan is not satisfied with just stopping us, though, he wants us to regress. I have seen some Christians excited and fired up about the things of God. They believe the Word of God is the answer. They sit in the front row at church with their Bible or Bible app open, and notepads ready to receive from God's Word service after service. Then suddenly, they are sitting in the back. One Sunday, I looked up and realize they are no longer coming to church.

They have allowed the enemy to impede their forward movement by bringing discouragement into their mind. Some circumstance has occurred in their life and the enemy whispers in their ear, "See, I told you it wouldn't work. Look where you are at now! You'll never succeed! It's just too hard! Why even bother trying?"

To discourage simply means that we allow someone or something to cause us to quit. Know what? That's the name of satan's game. If the enemy can get us to quit thinking we can win, we take ourselves out of the game. The enemy wants to pressure us until we throw up our hands and quit. We lose our peace and start warring against ourselves, our family and friends, and others who would support and encourage us.

I have battled and warred against discouragement. For years, I would go to bed, tears running down my face, crying like a baby because it just seemed like nothing was working...

like God wasn't coming through...

    like nothing was happening as it should...

        like every plan would fail... every hope would expire.

I knew God had spoken to me and had given me a vision, but it seemed like it wasn't coming to pass. However, I kept refusing to give up. Every morning, I'd wake up and feel like I could go on.

**At times, we look at our circumstances
and are tempted to become discouraged,
but God was showing me
it was going to look better every morning.
Yes, His mercies are new every morning!**

Warnings from Israel's History

We are going to learn some things about dealing with discouragement as we read 1 Corinthians 10:1-11. We have a summary of the Israelites in the wilderness after they left Egypt. They are headed to the Promised Land which God told them was a land flowing with milk and honey. The Promised Land represented their vision, but they found themselves in the wilderness. We are going to look at their journey in the wilderness and discuss the causes of their discouragement and the cures to overcome that discouragement.

Moreover, brethren, I would not that you should be ignorant how that all our fathers were under the cloud, and all passed through the sea. And were all baptized unto Moses in the cloud in the sea; And did all eat the same spiritual meat. And did all drink the same spiritual drink; for they drank of that spiritual Rock that followed them; And that rock was Christ. But with many of them God was not well pleased; for they were overthrown in the wilderness. (Verses 1-5 KJV)

When the vision God has shown us doesn't occur right away, don't be overthrown and overcome like the Israelites

were. Go on to the Promised Land even though we must go through a wilderness experience first. It's our right and privilege in Christ to complete our journey.

- *Don't be satisfied with being saved from Egypt.*
- *Refuse to settle for just coming out of bondage. Go all the way into the Promised Land.*
- *Reject discouragement. Embrace the boldness and courage of the Lord.*
- *Decide to be a victor not a victim.*
- *Renew your mind with the truth.* **Confess***: "God's plans for me are good, not evil, giving me a hopeful future."*

"Now these things were examples, to the intent that we should not lust after evil things, as they also lusted." **[In other words, don't do what they did.]** *"Neither be ye idolaters, as were some of them; as it is written, the people sat down to eat and drink, and they rose up to play. Neither let us commit fornication, as some of them committed, and fell in one day three and twenty thousand. Neither let us tempt Christ, as some of them also tempted, and were destroyed of serpents. Neither murmur ye, as some of them also murmured, and were destroyed of the destroyer. Now all these things happened unto them for examples* **[so we'll know what not to do]***: and they are written for our admonition* **[our warning]***, upon whom the ends of the world are come. Wherefore let him that thinketh he standeth, take heed lest he fall. There hath no temptation taken you but such as is common to man: but God is faithful..."* (1 Corinthians 10:6-13 KJV emphasis added)

Remember,
God is faithful.

That's what I can declare right now. After all those years of struggling, I can honestly say God is faithful. I want you to know, even when it seemed like it was not working, right in the midst of that trouble, the Lord spoke to me and said, "Just because it seems like it's not working, does not mean that it's not." In other words, He was saying, "Don't give up."

There has no temptation taken you, but such as is common to man, but God is faithful who will not suffer you to be tempted above that ye are able; but will with the temptation also make a way to escape, that ye may be able to bear it. (Verse 13 KJV)

You can bear what you're going through, so don't give up!

Complaining Is Not Going to Help You

*Soon the people began to **complain** about their hardship, and the LORD **heard everything they said**. Then the LORD's **anger blazed against them**, and he sent a fire to rage among them, and he destroyed some of the people in the outskirts of the camp. Then the people screamed to Moses for help, and when he prayed to the LORD, the fire stopped. After that, the area was known as Taberah (which means "the place of burning"), because fire from the LORD had burned among them there. **Then the foreign rabble who were traveling with the Israelites began to crave the good things of Egypt. And the people of Israel also began to complain.** "Oh, for some meat!" they exclaimed. "We remember the fish we used to eat for free in Egypt. And we had all the cucumbers, melons, leeks, onions, and garlic we wanted. But now our appetites are gone. All we ever see is this manna!" (Numbers 11:1-6 NLT)*

It says when the people complained, it displeased, angered, and grieved the Lord. When Moses prayed, the fire was quenched. However, then in verse 4, it says there were non-Jews among them who began to want what they left behind in Egypt (the world). These were disgruntled, discontented, negative, unhappy people. When the children of Israel listened to these negative people, they began to complain again, too. We must watch our associations, or they will start to discourage us.

Proverbs 22:24 says, "Don't hang out with angry people; don't keep company with hotheads. Bad temper is contagious—don't get infected." (MSG)

The Bible says don't associate with angry, disgruntled, unhappy, discontented people. Don't hang out with people who are always murmuring, complaining, and always looking for the negative in situations. We're supposed to separate from those people because if we keep hanging with folks like them, suddenly, we're angry, complaining, and focusing on the negative, too.

It will be discouraging to be around those people because they will point out any little flaw in our dreams and ideas. The Bible says not to cast our pearls before swine and don't give that which is Holy to the dogs (Matthew 7:6).

Our vision, our dreams, and our goals are precious to us. We can't share them with people who don't value them.

Negative, murmuring people focus on what they don't have, much like those who complained saying, "We remember the fish we used to eat for free in Egypt." That's a lie, nothing was free in Egypt. They worked from sunup to sundown and didn't get a penny. If we listen to the devil, he will tell us the world was better.

Then, **Moses heard the people complaining and became discouraged.** We must be cautious about who we listen to and guard our ears, or we will risk becoming discouraged, too.

> *So Moses said to the Lord, "Why have You afflicted Your servant? And why have I not found favor in Your sight, that You have laid the burden of all these people on me? Did I conceive all these people? Did I beget them, that You should say to me, 'Carry them in your bosom, as a guardian carries a nursing child,' to the land which You swore to their fathers? Where am I to get meat to give to all these people? For they weep all over me, saying, 'Give us meat, that we may eat.' I am not able to bear all these people alone, because the burden is too heavy for me. If You treat me like this, please kill me here and now—if I have found favor in Your sight—and do not let me see my wretchedness!"* (Numbers 11:11-15 NKJV)

That's the language of discouragement.

I feel like giving up.	I want to quit.
I've had it.	Somebody else can do it.
I don't want to get out of bed.	I don't want to go to work.
The Word is not working for me.	What difference does it make?
I studied. I prayed. I've done everything I know to do.	Now, I'm all by myself.
Nobody cares about me.	Nobody is going through what I'm going though.

So the Lord said to Moses: "Gather to Me seventy men of the elders of Israel, whom you know to be the elders of the people and officers over them; bring them to the tabernacle of meeting, that they may stand there with you. (Verse 16, NKJV)

Moses had people around him who were both willing and qualified to serve with him, but his focus was on the complainers. Oftentimes, the resources are present, as are those who care about us, but we are so focused on the naysayers, those who tell us we can't do it, that we don't notice the resources all around us.

**Overcome discouragement
by seeking God daily.**

If we are going to overcome discouragement, we need to turn to God and keep His Word in front of us. When we do, we will be amazed at how the Holy Spirit will give us encouragement. We must have a daily quiet time. It's not the length of it. It's the consistency of it.

Moses told God he couldn't handle that situation. When we go to God, He will give us encouragement and a strategy. In Numbers 13:1-3, "And the LORD spoke to Moses, saying, 'Send men to spy out the land of Canaan, which I am giving to the children of Israel; from each tribe of their fathers you shall send a man, every one a leader among them.' So Moses sent them from the Wilderness of Paran according to the command of the LORD, all of them men who *were* heads of the children of Israel" (NKJV).

Twelve men were sent out to spy on the land. God had told them He had given them the land, but planning is our responsibility. God gives us the victory, but it's our responsibility to plan. They returned after 40 days with an account of what they saw.

*Now they departed and came back to Moses and Aaron
and all the congregation of the children of Israel in the*

*Wilderness of Paran, at Kadesh; they brought back word to them and to all the congregation and showed them the fruit of the land. Then they told him, and said: "We went to the land where you sent us. It truly flows with milk and honey, and this is its fruit. Nevertheless the people who dwell in the land are strong; the cities are fortified and very large; moreover we saw the descendants of Anak there. The Amalekites dwell in the land of the South; the Hittites, the Jebusites, and the Amorites dwell in the mountains; and the Canaanites dwell by the sea and along the banks of the Jordan." Then Caleb quieted the people before Moses, and said, "Let us go up at once and take possession, for we are well able to overcome it." But the men who had gone up with him said, **"We are not able to go up against the people, for they are stronger than we." And they gave the children of Israel a bad report of the land** which they had spied out, saying, "The land through which we have gone as spies is **a land that devours its inhabitants**, and all the people whom we saw in it are men of great stature. There we saw the giants (the descendants of Anak came from the giants); **and we were like grasshoppers in our own sight, and so we were in their sight.*** (Numbers 13:26-33 NKJV emphasis added)

Ten of the twelve spies were discouraged by what they saw because they judged the opposition, the problems, and the challenges by their personal resources and abilities. It's evident in their fearful, negative language. **Whenever we measure the opposition, the problems, and the challenges by our own personal ability and resources, it will discourage us.**

However, Joshua and Caleb did the opposite. They saw the same giants, and fortified cities, but they measured the opposition, the problems, and the challenges by God's promise and His ability. "With God on our side, they said, we are well able to handle it." We have to be careful who we listen to.

In Numbers 14:1-4, the story continues. The Israelites gravitated towards the negative report instead of the positive report and began to cry and whisper among themselves.

> *So all the congregation lifted up their voices and cried, and the people wept that night. And all the children of Israel complained against Moses and Aaron, and the whole congregation said to them, "If only we had died in the land of Egypt! Or if only we had died in this wilderness! Why has the Lord brought us to this land to fall by the sword, that our wives and children should become victims? Would it not be better for us to return to Egypt?" So they said to one another, "Let us select a leader and return to Egypt." (NKJV)*

They listened to the wrong people, became discouraged, and desired to return to Egypt - the very place where they had been delivered. **Because of a negative report, they forgot about what God had already done for them and dismissed what He had promised them.**

**Choosing to believe what others tell us
instead of what God has said
can cause delays in the purpose
that God has for our lives.**

When the people **chose** to listen to the wrong people instead of Joshua and Caleb, they brought about a 40-year delay in entering the Promised Land God had already given them. It was self-sabotage.

All those years when I was struggling, I began to seek His face, read and study His Word, and pray for God's wisdom. Philippians 1:6 says, "Being confident of this very thing, that He who has begun a good work in you will complete *it* until the day of Jesus Christ" (NKJV). **We all experience delays, and we all experience detours on** the way to the fulfillment of our vision. We need to keep in mind, God started this work in us, and He'll finish it.

Discouragement Is a Spirit

Discouragement is not just an emotion. Discouragement is a demonic, evil, and hateful spirit that attacks us to make us give up. **It is an enemy to our inner peace and an enemy to our assignment.** We're in a spiritual war. Ephesians 6:12 says we aren't fighting flesh and blood, but against principalities, powers, rulers of the darkness of this world, and spiritual wickedness in heavenly places. James 4:7 tells us to submit ourselves to God and if we resist the devil, he will flee from us. If we don't submit to the revelation of Scripture and resist, that demon of discouragement will drive us to the ground.

The goal of satan is to steal, kill, and destroy us. He's ruthless and wants us out of the way. There were times I would be so discouraged, it felt like a heavy cloud was on me. I could almost feel it. It took me years to find out that it's a spirit. Oftentimes, we think it's just us. We think it's just an emotion, but we're dealing with a spirit. We need to learn how to use the weapons of spiritual warfare God has given us in His Word and resist the enemy.

An Example of What Not to Do

Looking at Israel in the wilderness teaches us what **not** to do when the enemy comes against us. We have a vision to go to our promised land. We want to walk in that abundant life, but there will always be people who are not going to have the same ambition, the same vision, the same dream, and the same desire to do any better. They will be satisfied with less than God's best. If we are not careful, they will discourage us.

> *Now the sons of Reuben and the sons of Gad had very large herds of cattle, and they saw the land of Jazer and the land of Gilead [on the east side of the Jordan River], and indeed, the place was suitable for raising livestock. So the sons of Gad and of Reuben came and spoke to Moses, to Eleazar the*

*priest, and to the leaders of the congregation, saying, "[The country around] Ataroth, Dibon, Jazer, Nimrah, Heshbon, Elealeh, Sebam, Nebo, and Beon, the land which the L*ORD* conquered before the congregation of Israel, is a land [suitable] for livestock, and your servants have [very large herds of] livestock." They said, "If we have found favor in your sight, let this land be given to your servants as a possession. Do not take us across the Jordan [River]." But Moses said to the sons of Gad and the sons of Reuben, "Shall your brothers go to war while you sit here? Now why are you discouraging the hearts of the Israelites from crossing over into the land which the L*ORD* has given them?"* (Numbers 32:1-7 AMP)

God promised the nation of Israel to bring them out of Egypt and bring them into the Promised Land, a land flowing with milk and honey. However, the tribes of Reuben and Gad got right there to the door of the Promised Land, and because they were herdsmen and the land was nice, **they were content to stay right where they were so they would not have to fight the inhabitants of the Promised Land.**

However, Moses said leaving them where they were would discourage the rest of them. He told these two tribes they needed to go over there and fight with the rest of the children of Israel. "Once we win," Moses told them, "if you want to come back over here, you can, but you're going to go over and fight with the rest of us." Therefore, **we need to be careful not to let others who don't really want to enter the Promise Land discourage us.**

We also need to be aware our journey to the Promised Land may be uncomfortable. Numbers 21:4 says, "They journeyed from mount Hor by the way of the Red sea, to compass the land of Edom. And the soul of the people was much discouraged…" (KJV). The Good News Translation says, "but on the way the people lost their patience." The Douay-Rheims 1899 American Edition says they "began to be weary of their journey and labour," and the Amplified Bible Classic Edition says, "the people became impatient, depressed, much discouraged because of the trials of the way." The route they were forced to take was a rough one, filled with sand, gravel, and rocks. There are going to be irritations, discomfort, and some trouble in our lives, but we can't allow them to discourage us.

Numbers 21:5 shows us what **not** to do. *"And the people **spoke against God and against Moses**, Why have you brought us out of Egypt to die in the wilderness? For there is no bread, neither is there any water, and **we loathe** this light (**contemptible, unsubstantial) manna"*(AMPC emphasis added).

When we have a challenge or a problem in life…

1. We shouldn't talk against God because He is on our side.
2. We shouldn't get angry at our spiritual leader either because they're there to help us get to our promised land.
3. We shouldn't despise God's Word (manna).
4. We should run to God and His Word.

If we read the rest of the story, those who complained and murmured were bitten by poisonous snakes. Whenever we get over into murmuring and complaining, we open the door for satan (snakes) to come into our life. God told Moses to get a pole and put a brass serpent on it which represents Jesus Christ overcoming satan on the cross. God said when a person is bitten, if they'll look up at the pole, they will live.

**Look to Jesus and you will live.
You will make it.**

›› ASK YOURSELF...

Am I discouraged? Have I been tempted to quit?

Has satan tried to dissuade me from getting in the Word, meditating on the Word, praying, witnessing, giving, or loving?

Have I been complaining?

›› APPLY WHAT YOU'VE LEARNED

Start to notice who you are hanging around. Are they angry, disgruntled, unhappy, discontented people? Are they always murmuring, complaining, and looking for the negative in situations? Make adjustments to these associations as needed.

CHAPTER 8

OVERCOME DISCOURAGEMENT WITH KEY REMEDIES

*"Behold my servant, [Jesus] whom I uphold; mine elect, in whom my soul delighteth. I have put my spirit upon him; he shall bring forth judgment to the Gentiles. He shall not cry, nor lift up, nor cause his voice to be heard in the street. A bruised reed shall he not break, and the smoking flax shall he not quench; he shall bring forth judgment unto truth. **He shall not fail nor be discouraged,** till he has set judgment in the earth: and the isles shall wait for his law."* (Isaiah 42:1-4 KJV emphasis added)

**Jesus won't fail,
and He won't be discouraged.
He is our example of what we should do!**

There are four keys to overcoming discouragement.

1. Have a Vision
2. Hold On to the Vision
3. Manage Our Emotions
4. Put Our Trust in God Only

Key #1: Have a Vision

The Bible says in Proverbs 29:18a, "Where there is no vision, the people perish…" (KJV). In her book, *Do Great Exploits: Say Yes to Your Dreams When It's Easier to Say No,* Michelle Johnson writes, "People perish without a vision. They remain as and where they are, and their purpose in life goes unfulfilled." I'm not talking about a dream we had at night or something mystical. I'm saying we need a goal, an ambition, a desire, and something we are shooting for in life. We all need to have something in our lives we are aiming to achieve.

Vision and hope are important because we can't have faith without them. Hebrews 11:1a says, "Now faith is the substance of things hoped for…" (KJV). Our faith gives substance to our vision. If we don't have hope, our faith has nothing to connect to and pray to receive. Mark 11:24 says, "Therefore I say to you, whatever things you ask when you pray, believe that you receive *them,* and you will have *them.*" (NKJV). We must have a vision and a desire before we can have faith to receive.

Jesus had a vision. In John 4:34, "Jesus saith unto them, my meat is to do the will of him that sent me and to finish his work" (KJV). In John 17:4, Jesus said, "I have glorified You on the earth. I finished the work which You have given Me to do" (NKJV). Jesus had a vision. He was headed somewhere. He had a plan to achieve what God had put in His heart, and He was moving in a certain direction.

God can't help us until we know what we want to achieve. James 1:6-8 says, "But when you ask for something, you must have faith and not doubt. Anyone who doubts is like an ocean wave tossed around in a storm. If you are that kind of person, you can't make up your mind, and you surely can't be trusted. So don't expect the Lord to give you anything at all" (CEV).

Key #2: Hold On to the Vision

Then the Lord answered me and said: Write the vision and make it plain on tablets, that he may run who reads it. For the vision is yet for an appointed time; But at the end it will speak, and it will not lie. Though it tarries, wait for it; Because it will surely come, it will not tarry. Behold the proud, His soul is not upright in him; But the just shall live by his faith. (Habakkuk 2:2-4 NKJV)

Discouragement comes in when our vision tarries (*delays*). Anything worthwhile in life is not going to happen overnight. Whether it's marriage, raising children, having a successful career, or getting a college degree, anything worthwhile in life takes time. Though it tarries, we are to wait for it. There are six things we need to do to successfully hold on to our vision.

First, write it down. I have a journal I've been keeping now for years. In this journal, I record the things God says to me, promises God makes to me, and things God says He wants me to do. God will give us a vision, but we are to write it down and keep it where we can see it.

Second, anticipate challenges. In John 16:33, Jesus says, "These things I have spoken to you, that in Me you may have peace. In the world you will have tribulation; but be of good cheer, I have overcome the world" (NKJV). Jesus said He has already overcome anything we are going to face. He'll show us how to overcome problems and distractions. Difficulty is going to come, so anticipate it. Then when it shows up, don't start doubting the dream.

Third, don't let the vision depart from your eyes. Proverbs 4:21 instructs us to not let God's Word depart from our eyes. Hebrews 12:2 says, "[**looking away from all that will distract us** and] focusing our eyes on Jesus, who is the Author and Perfecter of faith [the first incentive for our belief and the One who brings our faith to maturity], who for the **joy [of accomplishing the goal]** set before Him endured the cross, disregarding the shame, and sat down at the right hand of the throne of God [revealing His deity, His authority, and the completion of His work]"(AMP emphasis added). In other words, Jesus endured whatever suffering came His way because He never let the vision depart from His eyes. When I feel discouragement coming on, I go to what He said, and I keep the vision in front of me. There are challenges, trials, and problems, but we must keep our vision in front of us. We cannot allow problems, challenges, and trouble to cloud our vision.

Fourth, edify, encourage, and build yourself up by praying in the Spirit. Jude 20 says, "But ye, beloved, building up yourselves on your most holy faith, praying in the Holy Ghost" (KJV). I spend quite a bit of time praying in the Spirit because sometimes an attack from the enemy comes into my mind. If I allow those thoughts to come into my mind, it shifts my focus from my vision. I just change gears and do not let my head dominate me. If I keep praying in the Spirit, my thoughts are going to line up.

Fifth, receive the comfort of God through His Holy Spirit. The Holy Spirit is on the inside of us. He wants us to win over any temptation and make it through every trial. 2 Corinthians 1:3-7 says, "Thank God, the Father of our Lord Jesus Christ, that he is our Father and the source of all mercy and comfort. For he gives us comfort in our trials so that we, in turn, may be able to give the same sort of strong sympathy to others in theirs. Indeed, experience shows that the more we share Christ's suffering the more we are able to give of his encouragement. This means that if we experience trouble we can pass on to you comfort and spiritual help; for if we ourselves have been comforted we know how to encourage you to endure patiently the same sort of troubles that we have ourselves endured. We are quite confident that if you have to suffer troubles as we have done, then, like us, you will find the comfort and encouragement of God" (PHILLIPS).

Sixth, make a determined decision not to quit. We must make the decision not to let satan or any trials and struggles make us quit. Refuse to give up. 2 Timothy 2:3 says, "You therefore must endure hardship as a good soldier of Jesus Christ" (NKJV). That means to hold on to that Word and refuse to surrender. It says **hold on, don't cave in, don't give up, endure.** Galatians 6:9 says, "Let us not be weary in well-doing for in due season, we shall reap, if we faint not" (KJV). The only thing that will keep us from reaping the vision is if we cave in, give up, and quit. That means winning is in our hands.

Key #3: Manage Our Emotions

In Luke 9:51-56 and Mark 3:1-7, Jesus teaches us why managing our emotions is so important. We're made in such a way that when negative stuff happens around us, it affects the way we feel on the inside. Whenever there's a disappointment, challenge, test, or trial, it makes us feel a certain way. In those moments, we must control our feelings and not allow those feelings to get us off track.

In Luke 9:51-56, Jesus went to a city in Samaria, but the Samaritans said, "We don't want you holding a meeting here." Peter, James, and John wanted to call fire down from heaven and burn them all up. Jesus wouldn't allow being rejected by the Samaritans to control Him. He kept His vision before Him and continued on toward Jerusalem.

In Mark 3:1-7, Jesus came upon a man who had a withered hand. Jesus asked the Pharisees if there was a law for healing on the Sabbath. No one answered. Jesus looked around among the crowd with anger because of the hardness of their hearts. They didn't care anything about that man with the withered hand. Jesus was angry, but He didn't allow His feelings to control Him. He healed the man. We must learn how to manage our feelings. Remember that self-control (temperance) is a fruit of the Holy Spirit. What we think about is going to affect our emotions. Therefore, to control our feelings, we must control our thoughts.

Don't keep thinking about how somebody hurt or disappointed you because that's going to affect your emotions and lead you into discouragement.

Key #4: Put Our Trust in God Only

John 2:24-25 says, "But Jesus didn't trust them, for he knew mankind to the core. **No one needed to tell him how changeable human nature is!" (TLB).**

The key to overcoming discouragement is not to put our trust in people because we're human. They will disappoint us. We need to put our trust in God only. That way, if somebody doesn't do what we think they should do or say what we think they should say or act the way we think they should act, it doesn't throw us off course.

›› ASK YOURSELF...

Do I have a vision for my life?

Have I been putting my trust in people instead of God?

How can I better control my emotions?

›› CONFESSION DURING TIMES OF DISCOURAGEMENT

I declare and decree Isaiah 41:10 over me right now. "Father, I'm not afraid for You are with me. I'm not dismayed because You're my God. You have strengthened me. You're helping me. You're upholding me with the right hand of righteousness." You've begun a good work in me, and You will finish it. I trust in You.

CHAPTER 9

SECURE VICTORY OVER DEPRESSION

I waited patiently for God to help me; then he listened and heard my cry. **He lifted me out of the pit of despair**, *out from the bog and the mire, and set my feet on a hard, firm path, and steadied me as I walked along. He has given me a new song to sing, of praises to our God.* **Now many will hear of the glorious things he did for me, and stand in awe before the Lord, and put their trust in him.** *Many blessings are given to those who trust the Lord and have no confidence in those who are proud or who trust in idols.* (Psalm 40:1-4 TLB emphasis added)

God wants us to be successful and wants us to use our success as a platform to win others to Him. To put it another way, others will see what the Lord has done for us and will trust and have faith in Him as well. Psalm 43:5 sheds light on depression.

"Why are you in despair, O my soul? And why are you restless and disturbed within me? Hope in God and wait expectantly for Him, for I shall again praise Him, The help of my [sad] countenance and my God." (AMP)

"Why are you cast down, O my soul?" (NKJV)

We are given the definition of depression, shown the battleground of depression is an inward situation, and supplied with the remedy for it in this verse.

The issue is not just what's happening around us that makes us depressed. It is how we respond. Notice depression will affect our appearance.

What is depression?

- To be depressed—*to be cast down, gloomy, and discouraged in our soul.*
- Pressed down and feeling bad about ourselves or our circumstances.
- A feeling of dejection and/or hopelessness.
- A place of loneliness and the pit of despair.
- A demonic attack seeking to destroy us.

Depression leads to a destiny of regression. The word *regress* means to retreat and move to a worst state. It is the opposite of progression and means to move back instead of advancing forward. Regression can be a result of a disappointment caused by dashed, shattered, ruined, or unfulfilled expectations. We expect to have a happy marriage. We expect to have happy, joyful, fulfilled, responsible children. We anticipate that our work will be rewarding and successful. When our expectations go unfulfilled, depression sets in.

All people experience unfulfilled expectations as a part of life. I've been disappointed in myself, in other people, and occasionally, we get disappointed in God. Disappointment oftentimes leads to discouragement. Discouragement is defined as being disheartened, dispirited, and characterized by a loss of drive, enthusiasm, and energy as well as an impediment to forward motion. Then, discouragement leads to the third phase, which is depression.

Disappointment > Discouragement > Depression

We need to understand what we're dealing with because a part of overcoming anything is to understand the war we are engaged in.

The first level is what I would call the **mildly depressed** person. This person feels sad because of a disappointment. Usually, this person wants to be alone. Their thoughts are usually negative, and this person has a sour attitude. At this level, simple adjustments can get a person out this mindset. For example, years ago, my daughter Tiffany played basketball in school. She was very intense. She would be disappointed if she missed the last shot, but by the time we got home, she would've made minor adjustments and would be asking what's for dinner. When we are mildly depressed, we can make minor adjustments and knock ourselves out of it.

Despondency, the next level, is a little worse than being mildly depressed. When we're mildly depressed, we may meditate on it or feel bad for a little while, but we soon want to return to the game. When we reach despondency, we think about quitting. Despondency leads to inactivity. We don't want to do anything.

Then, there's a third level called **despair** which means *to be utterly without a way and without a resource*. It means *a total loss of hope*. This prompts reckless actions or violence in the face of defeat or frustration. Oftentimes, this is the place where people attempt to kill themselves. The enemy jumps in and plants seeds in their thoughts like, "You might as well take your life. Why don't you just kill yourself?"

[Warning: If you are having suicidal thoughts, please seek help immediately. National Suicide Prevention Lifeline 1-800-273-TALK (8255) or text the Crisis Text Line (text HELLO to 741741).]

What are the characteristics of depression?

1. Hopelessness, despair, sadness, apathy
2. A loss of perspective; Everything becomes colorless, drab
3. A change in physical activity, eating, and sleeping habits
4. General loss of self-esteem
5. Withdrawal from others, fear of rejection, running away, suicide
6. Over-sensitive to what others say and touchy
7. Difficulty in handling anger and other emotions
8. Overwhelming sense of guilt that may be real or imagined
9. Driven to alcoholism, drugs, other escapes
10. Dependency projected upon others

Examples of Prevalent Causes of Depression

#1 Events:
- Death of a child, spouse, parent, sibling, friend
- Major financial problems
- Business failure
- Termination from a job
- Unwanted pregnancy
- Divorce
- Debilitating accident
- Unemployment
- Jail sentence
- Extramarital affair
- Academic failure
- Sexual, physical, or emotional abuse

#2 Biological or Psychological Factors:
- Disease/illness
- Chronic conditions
- Heart disease
- Diabetes

- Chronic pain
- Thyroid conditions
- Anxiety disorders
- Generalized depression
- Bipolar
- Schizophrenia
- Brain chemistry imbalance

#3 Side Effects of Drugs or Medications
- Prescriptions
- Drug interactions
- Illegal drugs
- Vitamin deficiency

#4 Rejection
- From a loved one
- From a family member
- From an employer or client
- From a friend or church member

#5 Failure of any Kind
- Job
- Parenting
- Marriage
- Finances
- Goals

#6 Unwise Comparison to Others
- Appearance
- Knowledge
- Possessions
- Status or their position in life
- Abilities

#7 Physical Behaviors
- Lack of nutrition
- Insufficient exercise
- Lack of sleep

#8 Social Behaviors
- Bullying in person
- Cyberbullying
- Gossip

#9 Self-Pity
- Feeling sorry for yourself
- Inward focus
- Believing no one else is in your situation or loves you

#10 Lack of Intimacy with God
- Lack of prayer life
- Decrease in spiritual development
- Lack of reading God's Word
- Blaming God

Rapport, Reassurance, Rest, Revelation, Reorganization

In 1 Kings 18, the prophet Elijah confronted the people of Israel about wicked King Ahab, his wife Jezebel, and the prophets of Baal (a god). They had led the people of Israel into idolatry. In 1 Kings 18:21, Elijah asked the people why they were wavering between two beliefs. He challenged them by saying, if God is God, serve God. If Baal is God, serve Baal, but don't waver from side to side, make a choice. Then, he issued a challenge to the 850 evil prophets of Baal to build an altar, put an ox on it but not to ignite the fire. He would also build an altar and sacrifice an ox. Then, they would both call on their god, and the god who answered by fire, would be considered the one true God. The 850 prophets pled and called on Baal all day, but there was no fire or manifestation of Baal.

Elijah dug a trench around his altar and then he said to bring him twelve barrels of water. He drenched the sacrifice and trench.

He called out to God, who sent fire from heaven that burned up the sacrifice, burned up the stones and the wood, and dried up all the water. He called out to the people of Israel and told them to kill all the evil prophets of Baal and destroy their altar. Then, he told Ahab to get back to his house because it was getting ready to rain. It hadn't rain for three and a half years, but suddenly, the sky grew dark, the wind came up, and it began pouring.

1 Kings 19:1-2 says, "When Ahab told Queen Jezebel what Elijah had done, and that he had slaughtered the prophets of Baal, she sent this message to Elijah: 'You killed my prophets, and now I swear by the gods that I am going to kill you by this time tomorrow night.'" (TLB). Though this man of God had just called fire down from heaven, he became afraid.

> *So Elijah fled for his life; he went to Beersheba, a city of Judah, and **left his servant there. Then he went on alone into the wilderness,** traveling all day, and sat down under a broom bush and prayed that he might die. "I've had enough," he told the Lord. "Take away my life. I've got to die sometime, and it might as well be now." Then he lay down and slept beneath the broom bush. But as he was sleeping, an Angel touched him and told him to get up and eat! He looked around and saw some bread baking on hot stones and a jar of water! So he ate and drank and lay down again. Then the Angel of the Lord came again and touched him and said, "Get up and eat some more, for there is a long journey ahead of you." So he got up and ate and drank, and the food gave him enough strength to travel forty days and forty nights to Mount Horeb, the mountain of God.* (1 Kings 19:3-8 TLB emphasis added)

Elijah had somebody close to him he could talk to, who was for him, and concerned about him, but he left his servant behind and went out by himself. That's always a problem. Instead of spending time with God and seeking His guidance and renewing his spiritual energy, he fled in fear. In the same way we can't go days without eating physical food, we can't go days without God's Word.

...But the Lord said to him, "What are you doing here, Elijah?" He replied, "I have worked very hard for the Lord God of the heavens; but the people of Israel have broken their covenant with you and torn down your altars and killed your prophets, and only I am left; and now they are trying to kill me too." "Go out and stand before me on the mountain," the Lord told him. And as Elijah stood there the Lord passed by, and a mighty windstorm hit the mountain; it was such a terrible blast that the rocks were torn loose, but the Lord was not in the wind. After the wind, there was an earthquake, but the Lord was not in the earthquake. And after the earthquake, there was a fire, but the Lord was not in the fire. And after the fire, there was the sound of a gentle whisper. When Elijah heard it, he wrapped his face in his scarf and went out and stood at the entrance of the cave.... Then the Lord told him, "Go back by the desert road to Damascus, and when you arrive, anoint Hazael to be king of Syria. Then anoint Jehu (son of Nimshi) to be king of Israel, and anoint Elisha (the son of Shaphat of Abel-meholah) to replace you as my prophet. Anyone who escapes from Hazael shall be killed by Jehu, and those who escape Jehu shall be killed by Elisha! And incidentally, there are 7,000 men in Israel who have never bowed to Baal nor kissed him!" So Elijah went and found Elisha who was plowing a field with eleven other teams ahead of him; he was at the end of the line with the last team. Elijah went over to him and threw his coat across his shoulders and walked away again. Elisha left the oxen standing there and ran after Elijah and said to him, "First let me go and say good-bye to my father and mother, and then I'll go with you!" Elijah replied, "Go on back! Why all the excitement?" Elisha then returned to his oxen, killed them,

and used wood from the plow to build a fire to roast their flesh. He passed around the meat to the other plowmen, and they all had a great feast. Then he went with Elijah, as his assistant. (1 Kings 19:9-21 TLB)

God delivered Elijah from depression by giving him the five basic needs of depressed people.

#1 Rapport: Depressed people need somebody to talk to who cares about and is concerned about them. Depressed people need to talk. They need a quiet, warm, accepting, firm person that's objective but not aggressive. Those depressed need to hear the truth spoken to them with love and compassion.

They need somebody who is warm, gentle, but can be firm. A depressed person needs to find somebody to talk to that they trust and they consider to be a spiritual person. This confidant could be a family member, friend, pastor, teacher, counselor, and/or therapist. Normally when people are under attack, the mistake they make is to run away from people, like Elijah left his servant and went out in the wilderness alone. God assured Elijah He was not alone.

#2 Reassurance: People who are depressed need reassurance, encouragement, confidence, and sometimes a boost in self-esteem. They need to be encouraged. They sometimes feel bad and worthless. They need a trusted friend to tell them they are strong and are going to make it. God told Elijah He had a purpose and a plan for his life.

#3 Rest: The depressed person needs rest. Elijah was tired physically, mentally, and emotionally. The lack of rest and sleep can cause any situation to worsen. God gave Elijah time to rest and protected him while he rested.

#4 Revelation: Elijah thought he was the only one serving God, but God revealed that He had 7,000 others so Elijah was not by himself. Those experiencing depression often feel like they are all alone and no one understands what they are going through.

#5 Reorganization: Elijah needed to reorganize his thoughts and his behavior. A depressed person needs to examine what they are thinking. They need to bring their thinking back in line with the Word of God because the Bible doesn't say they are worthless or a failure. God told Elijah he was not worthless, he was still going to serve Him, and still had a purpose to fulfill. Then, God gave him an assignment. There was life after depression.

Six Keys to Overcoming Depression

1. Pray
2. Control Emotions
3. Choose to Be Happy
4. Rejoice
5. Encourage Ourselves in the Lord
6. Submit to God

Key #1: Pray

The Bible says when we have pressure on us, when we are facing a temptation, a test, or a trial and feel depression coming on us, the first thing we need to do is pray in the Spirit. When we don't know how to pray, we ask the Holy Spirit to help us to pray.

> *And in the same way—by our faith—**the Holy Spirit helps us with our daily problems and in our praying. For we don't even know what we should pray for nor how to pray as we should**, but the Holy Spirit prays for us with such feeling that it cannot be expressed in words. And the Father who knows all hearts knows, of course, what the Spirit is saying as he pleads for us in harmony with God's own will.* (Romans 8:26-27 TLB emphasis added)

Then, we also need to pray with *our understanding* which means praying in our regular language while specifically praying about our situation and asking God for wisdom.

Dear brothers, is your life full of difficulties and temptations? Then be happy, for when the way is rough, your patience has a chance to grow. So let it grow, and don't try to squirm out of your problems. For when your patience is finally in full bloom, then you will be ready for anything, strong in character, full and complete. **If you want to know what God wants you to do, ask him, and he will gladly tell you, for he is always ready to give a bountiful supply of wisdom to all who ask him; he will not resent it.** *But when you ask him, be sure that you really expect him to tell you, for a doubtful mind will be as unsettled as a wave of the sea that is driven and tossed by the wind; and every decision you then make will be uncertain, as you turn first this way and then that. If you don't ask with faith, don't expect the Lord to give you any solid answer.* (James 1:2-8 TLB emphasis added)

Key #2: Control Emotions

The Psalmist is talking to his soul in Psalm 43:5. Remember, the soul is our mind, will, and emotions. Depression is attacking our mind and emotions, but we can take command over them! When bad things happen, we can develop negative feelings on the inside of us. If we want to control our emotions, we must change our thoughts and focus on the positive, not the negative.

We take control by speaking to our soul and declaring, "Soul, you are not going to be depressed, in Jesus' name."

Key #3: Choose to Be Happy

Psalm 118:24 says, "This is the day which the Lord hath made; we will rejoice and be glad in it" (KJV). We are a spirit, and we have a soul (our mind, emotions, and our will). Our will is our decision-maker.

We can make a decision and choose to stay happy and not focus on the negative. We can become acclimated to being depressed. We can choose depression and come to a place where depression is the way of life. However, we can choose to be happy and make that our way of life. We always have a choice.

NOTE: If you have changed your thinking and are still experiencing symptoms of depression, please seek a consultation with a healthcare practitioner to ensure you do not have an underlying medical condition that needs to be addressed.

Key #4: Rejoice

Isaiah 61:3a says, "To all who mourn in Israel he will give: beauty for ashes; joy instead of mourning; praise instead of heaviness..." (TLB). The remedy for the spirit of heaviness is to praise God. When I am feeling depressed, I put on the garment of praise. In Acts 16:22-26 it says, when the magistrates had laid many stripes upon Paul and Silas, they put them in prison, and put their feet in the stocks. Despite their situation, they chose to sing praises to God in the jail cell, and the other prisoners heard them.

Suddenly, there was a great earthquake so that the foundation of the prison was shaken. All the prison doors were open, and everyone's bands were loosed. God is worthy of praise and His worth has absolutely nothing to do with our circumstances. When we understand that principle, we can lift our hands up, rejoice, and praise Him no matter what issues we are facing in life.

**A merry heart does good, like medicine,
But a broken spirit dries the bones.
Proverbs 17:22 (NKJV)**

Key #5: Encourage Ourselves in the Lord

We can't wait for somebody else to encourage us. We need to encourage ourselves, talk to ourselves, and spend time talking to God. God wants us to get to a place in our Christian experience where we can go directly to Him. We have to encourage ourselves in the Lord because He knows exactly what we need. Remember, Isaiah 55:8 says, "'For my thoughts are not your thoughts, neither are your ways my ways,' saith the LORD" (KJV).

Key #6: Submit to God

James 4:7 says we are to submit to what God says and then resist the devil. We must speak to the spirit of depression and refuse to accept it in our lives and speak the name of Jesus over our situation! Nobody can do that for us.

> *Don't you yet understand? Don't you know by now that the everlasting God, the Creator of the farthest parts of the earth, never grows faint or weary?* **No one can fathom the depths of his understanding. He gives power to the tired and worn out, and strength to the weak.** *Even the youths shall be exhausted, and the young men will all give up. But* **they that wait upon the Lord shall renew their strength.** *They shall mount up with wings like eagles; they shall run* **and not be weary**; *they shall walk and not faint.* (Isaiah 40:28-31 TLB emphasis added)

2 Corinthians 4:8 says, "We are pressed on every side by troubles, but not crushed and broken. We are perplexed because we don't know why things happen as they do, but we don't give up and quit" (TLB).

Psalm 43:5 says, "O my soul, why be so gloomy and discouraged? Trust in God! I shall again praise him for his wondrous help; he will make me smile again, *for he is my God!*" (TLB).

›› ASK YOURSELF...

Do I display any of these characteristics of depression?
Have I isolated myself from others?

›› APPLY WHAT YOU'VE LEARNED

1. Pray
2. Control Your Emotions
3. Choose to Be Happy
4. Rejoice
5. Encourage Yourself in the Lord
6. Submit to God

NOTE: If you have applied the principles from this chapter and are still experiencing symptoms of depression, please seek a consultation with a healthcare practitioner to ensure you do not have an underlying medical condition that needs to be addressed.

CHAPTER 10

RESPOND EFFECTIVELY TO FEELINGS OF REJECTION

The actress Marilyn Monroe had fame and beauty. However, she committed suicide. A famous remark by her was, "Sometimes I feel my life has been one big rejection." At some point in our lives, we all must deal with rejection. It's hard to avoid because sometimes it's our own doing, but many times it's unrelated to anything we did wrong. Either way, the feeling of rejection can be the same. Even Jesus was rejected. The good news is that the Word of God shows us the key to overcoming rejection. However, first, let's get an understanding of rejection and explore its possible causes.

Rejection {def}:
- To be cast aside
- To be thrown away as having no value
- To not be wanted, accepted, or loved

Rejection Due to Our Own Behavior or Sin

Now the man Adam knew Eve as his wife, and she conceived and gave birth to Cain, and she said, "I have obtained a man (baby boy, son) with the help of the Lord.*" And [later] she gave birth to his brother Abel. Now Abel kept the flocks [of sheep and goats], but Cain cultivated the ground. And in the course of time Cain brought to the* Lord *an offering of the fruit of the ground. But Abel brought [an offering of] the [finest] firstborn of his flock and the fat portions. And the* Lord *had respect (regard) for Abel and for his offering; but for Cain and his offering He had no respect. So Cain became extremely angry (indignant), and he looked annoyed and hostile. And the* Lord *said to Cain, "Why are you so angry? And why do you look annoyed? If you do well [believing Me and doing what is acceptable and pleasing to Me], will you not be accepted?* **And if you do not do well [but ignore My instruction]**, *sin crouches at your door; its desire is for you [to overpower you], but you must master it." Cain talked with Abel his brother [about what God had said]. And when they were [alone, working] in the field, Cain attacked Abel his brother and killed him.* (Genesis 4:1-8 AMP)

Hebrews 11:4 says, "By faith Abel offered to God a more acceptable sacrifice than Cain, through which it was testified of him that he was righteous (upright, in right standing with God), and God testified by accepting his gifts. And though he died, yet through [this act of] faith he still speaks" (AMP).

That leads me to believe God gave Abel and Cain instructions concerning the offering. Abel obeyed the instructions, but Cain, through self-will, brought the offering he wanted to bring. The key to acceptance would have been to simply do what God told him to do. Sometimes, we experience rejection because of our own behavior, our own sin, or our own negligence.

Rejection Due to Weakness, Meanness, Failure, Negligence, Insensitivity, Sin in Others

So David went out wherever Saul sent him, and he acted wisely and prospered; and Saul appointed him over the men of war. And it pleased all the people and also Saul's servants. As they were coming [home], when David returned from killing the Philistine, the women came out of all the cities of Israel, singing and dancing, to meet King Saul with tambourines, [songs of] joy, and musical instruments. The women sang as they played and danced, saying, "Saul has slain his thousands, and David his ten thousands." Then Saul became very angry, for this saying displeased him; and he said, "They have ascribed to David ten thousand, but to me they have ascribed [only] thousands. Now what more can he have but the kingdom?" **Saul looked at David with suspicion [and jealously] from that day forward.**
(1 Samuel 18:5-9 AMP emphasis added)

David was rejected by Saul. When Saul got into rebellion, it opened the door for an evil spirit to oppress him and he tried to kill David. **David did nothing wrong.** Sometimes, people are rejected due to weakness, meanness, failure, negligence, insensitivity, or sin in others. It can be extremely painful to experience rejection because of others.

Rejection Due to Problems Unrelated to Us

If others have problems unrelated to us, we can make all the adjustments in the world, but it's not going to change them or that situation. Rather than realizing that other people may be dealing with issues unrelated to us (e.g., insecurities, trauma), we turn inward and become frustrated. We attempt to determine what's wrong with us when we haven't done anything wrong.

Rejection From Seeds Sown into Us as Children

Years ago, I was struggling big time emotionally and didn't have a clue what was wrong with me. When I asked the Lord what was wrong with me, He gave me one word: rejection. If anyone had asked me what my problem was, I never would have said rejection. In fact, I would have called it frustration.

Causes of Childhood Rejection

- **An Unwanted Pregnancy:** If we keep saying we don't want this child, we sow the seeds of rejection in the child before the child is even born.
- **An Abortion:** An attempt to abort a child can cause rejection.
- **Wrong Gender:** If we wanted a boy and got a girl, or a girl and got a boy. As the child grows up, they may feel rejected by the parents.
- **Born with learning or physical disabilities:** Because the child may not look or behave like others, this could lead to rejection by others.
- **Comparison Among Siblings:** When we were young, my godmother used to compare my godbrother to me. Every time he did anything wrong, she would tell him he needed to be more like me. Things like this can cause feelings of rejection. When siblings are compared to each other, no one wins.
- **Perceived Favoritism:** Although a parent may not be doing it on purpose, there may be instances where it appears they are favoring one of their children over the other. For instance, if dad attends the son's sporting events, but not the daughter's spelling bee. Grandparents, aunts, uncles, and even family friends need to realize how this can affect sibling and cousin relationships. It can plant seeds of rejection.
- **Lack of Parental Quality Time:** If parents work all the time and don't spend much time with their children, the child could grow up thinking they don't care about them or love them. It can lead to feelings of being unwanted.
- **Divorce:** Even though it is not usually the intent of parents who divorce to blame their children, often their children

internalize their parents' conflict and experience the seeds of rejection.

- **Peer Rejection:** Children and teenagers can reject each other due to peer pressure.
- **Unfaithful Spouse:** A spouse may feel rejected if their spouse has a physical or emotional affair with someone else.
- **Rejection from Children:** Our children can reject us even if we are doing everything we know to do.

The Fruits of the Seed of Rejection:

- rebellion
- anger
- bitterness
- guilt
- inferiority
- escapism- drugs, alcohol, television, work, social media
- judgmentalism
- poverty
- fear
- hopelessness
- defensiveness
- hardness
- distrust
- perfectionism
- disrespect
- competition
- jealousy

Cure for Rejection

The cure for rejection is security in Christ.

In Ephesians 3:14-17, the Apostle Paul is praying a prayer for the church at Ephesus. "For this cause, I bow my knees unto the Father of our Lord Jesus Christ, of whom the whole family in heaven and earth is named, that he would grant you, according to the riches of his glory, to be strengthened with might by his spirit in the inner man; that Christ may dwell in your hearts by faith; that ye being rooted and grounded in love" (KJV).

The Amplified Bible Classic Edition reads, "may you be rooted deep in love and founded securely on love" (Verse 17). He's using *rooted* which is biological terminology. He's also using *founded* which is architectural terminology. Rooted like a tree, but grounded, or founded, or established like a building. A tree must have a strong root system and a building must have a good foundation to withstand any kind of storm.

A strong root system and a good foundation is needed to withstand any storm.

Paul is praying they would be rooted like a tree and founded like a building in Christ's love. If a root of rejection sets up in our lives and we don't know how to break it, we just go from one incident of rejection to another incident of rejection to another incident of rejection. It will follow us for the rest of our lives. We should determine how to uproot it and get it out of our lives.

We must dig deep and discover what it means to be **securely** rooted and founded on Christ's love. Security is...

- a personal sense of worth, value, and well-being.
- a gift from God of freedom from fear, anxiety, doubt, or danger.
- a feeling of stability, safety, and confidence.
- a mindset of being safe and secure in the arms of the Almighty.

We experience frustration, a sense of failure, and a feeling of unfulfillment because we are rooted in the wrong thing. It is possible to be saved and yet not be firmly rooted and founded in God's love. It is difficult to stand against the storms of rejection and persecution without a strong root system and foundation.

I experienced rejections and persecution when I started to teach the Word of God. I thought everybody would be happy and receive what I was teaching. One of the best things that ever happened to me was to get persecuted early in ministry. I had to turn only to God for my security. Then when the Lord led me into various assignments, I was able to deal with persecution and rejection, knowing my assignment was to obey and please Him. He would take care of the rest.

> *Cursed is the one who trusts in man, who draws strength from mere flesh and whose heart turns away from the LORD. That person will be like a bush in the wastelands; they will not see prosperity when it comes. They will dwell in the parched places of the desert, in a salt land where no one lives.* ***But blessed is the one who trusts in the Lord, whose confidence is in him.*** *They will be like a tree planted by the water that sends out its roots by the stream. It does not fear when heat comes; its leaves are always green. It has no worries in a year of drought and never fails to bear fruit.* (Jeremiah 17:5-8 NIV emphasis added)

When we are rooted in the right thing, the drought can come, and we will not fear or fail. Rejection and people not approving and not accepting us is a drought.

**When we are rooted in God, it doesn't matter
when people don't respond or act
the way we think they should act.
We can still be productive and still yield fruit.**

In my senior year of college, I played basketball. I made an idol of it. It was the last game of the season, and they'd normally honor the seniors. I said something I shouldn't have said, and the coach kept me out of the game. Everybody played except me. I was humiliated and let it uproot my confidence, but I learned from my mistakes. Now, I put my confidence only in God.

Check Your Foundation

"Therefore everyone who hears these words of mine and puts them into practice is like a wise man who built his house on the rock. ***The rain came down, the streams rose, and the winds blew and beat against that house; yet it did not fall, because it had its foundation on the rock.*** *But everyone who hears these words of mine and does not put them into practice is like a foolish man who built his house on sand. The rain came down, the streams rose, and the winds blew and beat against that house, and it fell with a great crash."* (Matthew 7:24-27 NIV emphasis added)

In fair weather, it looks like both houses were founded on the same thing. However, the person who built their foundation on God's Word will see a difference when the weather changes in their life. A young woman called me and said, "I'm in a spiritual battle." I said to her, "You are a strong woman of God, keep standing on that Word."

We learn what we are really founded on when trouble, tribulation, challenges, tests, trials, or adversity comes into our lives.

Are we "founded" on the "rock" of God's Word and His love? Are we firmly established on the right foundation or is our validation in life built upon the "sand" of other sources of security?

The Sand Foundation

The sand foundation could be a job. If our job gives us a personal sense of worth, value, well-being, and provides a sense of security and safety, our life could come crashing down if the job is no longer there. Whatever our security is could be our sand foundation.

It's a very serious issue for some teenagers when their security is in a high school or college team sport. They feel they have to make the team to establish their sense of worth and value. There are those who are fortunate enough to get drafted, but if they build everything around this, when it doesn't happen, they are in trouble.

Maybe our whole system of validation and security is built around a relationship. We want somebody to love us. Teenagers are not stable enough to have a serious relationship. They don't understand that they do not have to have somebody else validate them. If they don't learn that, they will go from relationship to relationship and from hurt to hurt. By the time they're adults and ready for marriage, they may have been hurt so many times that they are full of rejection. When we are secure in ourselves, nobody can just come along and try to fill us with false security. Our security should be in God's love.

A sand foundation could be our financial status, our education, our looks, or the label inside of our clothes. It could be the car we drive, the kind of house we own, or the neighborhood in which we reside.

A sand foundation could be getting married. We may feel unwanted, or unloved because we don't have a spouse. We cannot look for a spouse to validate us or make us feel important. If we do, we are in for a rude awakening.

Also, our sense of worth, well-being, satisfaction, and happiness cannot be tied to our children, either. What are we going to do when they grow up and move away?

If our security is in people and what they think about us, we need to remember, there are some people who have problems that are unrelated to us.

We need to get to a place where we don't need any of these things or people to give us security and a sense of self-worth. Our foundation needs to be built on the "rock"—Christ.

God wants us to put our trust and security in Him rather than in other things or people, and then He'll utilize those things to bless us. When we become secure in Him, people can say whatever they will, and it doesn't bother us. It's just like water rolling off a duck's back.

The Rejection of Jesus

We despised him and rejected him—a man of sorrows, acquainted with bitterest grief. We turned our backs on him and looked the other way when he went by. He was despised, and we didn't care. (Isaiah 53:3 TLB emphasis added)

Isaiah 53:3 is somewhat of a summary of the life of Jesus. It says He was despised and rejected by men. That's not talking about one incident. This was a serious rejection.

That was the true light which shines upon every man as he comes into the world. He came into the world—the world he had created—and the world failed to recognize him. He came into his own creation, and his own people would not accept him. Yet wherever men did accept him he gave them the power to become sons of God. These were the men who truly believed in him, and their birth depended not on the course of nature nor on any impulse or plan of man, but on God. (John 1:11 PHILLIPS emphasis added)

If they would not accept Him, then that meant they rejected Him. None of us have ever experienced the kind of rejection Jesus experienced. How did Jesus deal with all this rejection and still complete His mission and His assignment? As we read through what Jesus experienced and how He handled rejection, I want each of us to put ourselves in His place and think about how we might handle each situation.

Jesus' Rejection in His Hometown

*He went to Nazareth, where he had been brought up, and on the Sabbath day he went into the synagogue, as was his custom. He stood up to read, and the scroll of the prophet Isaiah was handed to him. Unrolling it, he found the place where it is written: "The Spirit of the Lord is on me, because he has anointed me to proclaim good news to the poor. He has sent me to proclaim freedom for the prisoners and recovery of sight for the blind, to set the oppressed free, to proclaim the year of the Lord's favor." Then he rolled up the scroll, gave it back to the attendant and sat down. The eyes of everyone in the synagogue were fastened on him. He began by saying to them, "Today this scripture is fulfilled in your hearing." All spoke well of him and were amazed at the gracious words that came from his lips. "Isn't this Joseph's son?" they asked. Jesus said to them, "Surely you will quote this proverb to me: 'Physician, heal yourself!' And you will tell me, 'Do here in your hometown what we have heard that you did in Capernaum.'" "Truly I tell you," he continued, **"no prophet is accepted in his hometown.** I assure you that there were many widows in Israel in Elijah's time, when the sky was shut for three and a half years and there was a severe famine throughout the land. Yet Elijah was not sent to any of them, but to a widow in Zarephath in the region of Sidon. And there were many in Israel with leprosy in the time of Elisha the prophet, yet not one of them was cleansed—only Naaman the Syrian." **All the people in the synagogue were furious when they heard this. They got up, drove him out of the town, and took him to the brow of the hill on***

which the town was built, in order to throw him off the cliff. (Luke 4:16-29 NIV emphasis added)

When Jesus went to Nazareth where He had been brought up, and began to tell them about His mission, at first, "All spoke well of him and were amazed at the gracious words that came from his lips." Then someone asked, "Isn't this Joseph's son?" In other words, "We know Him and His family. What gives Him the authority to speak this way?"

We want to help the people in our family and community. However, when we tell them we have an assignment and are anointed by God, and they get angry and reject us like what happened to Jesus, how do we handle it?

Jesus' Rejection After He Heals the Demon-Possessed Man

In Luke 8:26-33, Jesus drove a legion of demons out of a man and sent them into a herd of pigs. The herd of pigs rushed down a steep bank and were drowned in the lake below. Everybody knew this demon-possessed man.

> *When those tending the pigs saw what had happened, they ran off and reported this in the town and countryside, and the people went out to see what had happened. When they came to Jesus, they found the man from whom the demons had gone out, sitting at Jesus' feet, dressed and in his right mind; and they were afraid. Those who had seen it told the people how the demon-possessed man had been cured.* ***Then all the people of the region of the Gerasenes asked Jesus to leave them because they were overcome with fear.*** *So he got into the boat and left.* (Luke 8:34-37 NIV emphasis added)

This man had been delivered, sat there fully clothed, and in his right mind. Yet, the people wanted Jesus to leave. They didn't want Him there. That's rejection.

Jesus' Rejection by the Religious Leaders

Jesus strictly warned them not to tell this to anyone. And he said, "The Son of Man must suffer many things and be rejected by the elders, the chief priests and the teachers of the law, and he must be killed and on the third day be raised to life." (Luke 9:21-22 NIV)

Jesus told His disciples He would be rejected by the elders, the chief priests, and the teachers of the Law. These three groups represented the religious establishment of His day. They were the religious authorities and supposedly had biblical knowledge of the coming Messiah. They were who the people looked up to, but Jesus was rejected by all of them. He had been given an assignment by God, anointed, and sent to bring healing and truth to God's people. Yet, the religious establishment didn't want anything to do with Him. In fact, they considered Jesus a cult leader.

Jesus' Rejection by the Samaritans

Jesus let nothing distract him from departing for Jerusalem because the time for him to be lifted up drew near, and he was full of passion to complete his mission there. So he sent messengers ahead of him as envoys to a village of the Samaritans. But as they approached the village, the people turned them away. They would not allow Jesus to enter, for he was on his way to worship in Jerusalem. (Luke 9:51-53 TPT)

Jesus' disciples were enraged at this rejection of Jesus. In fact, they wanted to call down fire from heaven and kill them all! Theirs was what we might call a more normal type of reaction to rejection. However, in verse 55, Jesus rebuked them sharply, saying, "Don't you realize what spews from your hearts when you say that? The Son of Man did not come to destroy life, but to bring life to the earth" (TPT).

Jesus' Rejection by His Followers

Jesus performed the miracle of the fish and the bread, and everybody had their bellies filled. A big crowd began to follow Him, but then He started preaching about commitment and suffering. He didn't change the prosperity message, He just added some commitment, some suffering, some holiness, and He added some self-denial to it. They didn't really like that part of the message. They liked the fish and the loaves message, but they didn't really care for the rest of the message.

> *"I am not like the bread your ancestors ate and later died. I am the living Bread that comes from heaven. Eat this Bread and you will live forever!"*
>
> *Jesus preached this sermon in the synagogue in Capernaum. And when many of Jesus' followers heard these things, it caused a stir. "That's disgusting!" they said. "How could anybody accept it?" And so from that time on* ***many of the disciples turned their backs on Jesus and refused to be associated with him.*** *(John 6:58-60, 66 TPT)*

Jesus went from feeding five thousand to offending five thousand.

> *So Jesus said to his twelve, "And you—do you also want to leave?" Peter spoke up and said, "But Lord, where would we go? No one but you gives us the revelation of eternal life. We're fully convinced that you are the Anointed One, the Son of the Living God, and we believe in you!" Then Jesus shocked them with these words: "I have hand-picked you to be my twelve, knowing that one of you is the devil." Jesus was referring to Judas Iscariot, son of Simon, for he knew that Judas, one of his chosen disciples, was getting ready to betray him. (John 6:67-71 TPT)*

Jesus was not only rejected by many of His followers, but He was also betrayed by one of His closest associates who had been traveling with Him for three years.

Jesus' Rejection by His Immediate Family

Then He went to a house [probably Peter's], but a throng came together again, so that Jesus and His disciples could not even take food. And when those who belonged to Him (His kinsmen) heard it, they went out to take Him by force, for they kept saying, He is out of His mind (beside Himself, deranged)! (Mark 3:20-21 AMPC)

Jesus was called and anointed to bring God's message to God's people, yet His immediate family not only didn't believe, but they rejected Him.

Jesus' Secret to Overcoming Rejection

How was Jesus able to overcome all this rejection without the negative results of rejection many people experience? We don't see anger or bitterness in these stories. He did not walk around hurt or full of self-pity. He didn't have a poor self-image. He didn't display loneliness or escapism. He's did not become judgmental and critical. He didn't put people down. He didn't stop praying. He wasn't disrespectful. He didn't defend Himself to be accepted.

> **If we can find out what His secret was, we can tap into it and overcome rejection in our own lives.**

*"I receive not glory from men [**I crave no human honor,** I look for no mortal fame], but I know you and recognize and understand that you have not the love of God in you. I have come in My Father's name and with His power, and you do not receive Me [**your hearts are not open to Me, you give Me no welcome**]; but if another comes in his own name and his own*

power and with no other authority but himself, you will receive him and give him your approval. How is it possible for you to believe [how can you learn to believe], you who [are content to seek and] receive praise and honor and glory from one another, and yet do not seek the praise and honor and glory which come from Him Who alone is God? (John 5:41-44 AMPC emphasis added)

Jesus wasn't looking for praise or validation from people. He was very secure in the fact His Father sent Him and loved Him (see John 8:29). Therefore, everything He did, His goal, His ambition, and His heart's desire was to please His Father.

**If we're trying to please folks and being rejected,
we should follow Jesus' example
and just focus on trying to please God.**

We can't obey the Spirit of God when we are concerned about others accepting us. We will never be able to follow God's assignment and answer God's call on our life if we are concerned about everybody validating us.

In John 16:32, Jesus told His disciples, "Indeed the hour is coming, yes, has now come, that you will be scattered, each to his own, and will leave Me alone. And yet I am not alone, because the Father is with Me" (NKJV). Jesus expressed no anger, no disappointment, and no hurt. The primary issue for Jesus was that His Father was there for Him. When we get that straight, we can take just about anything anybody says because our validation is not coming from them. If they are with us, fine, but if they're not with us, fine. If they talk good about us, fine, but if they talk bad about us, we don't have to give what they say any thought. We have to get to that place in order to walk with the Lord. When we do, nobody can stop us from fulfilling God's assignment in our life because we are obeying God.

Rooted and Grounded in God's Love: The Key to Overcoming Rejection

Jesus was grounded in God's love. That's the key to overcoming rejection. There are three things we must be rooted in concerning God's love.

The Lord appeared from of old to me [Israel], saying, Yes, I have loved you with an everlasting love; therefore with loving-kindness have I drawn you and continued My faithfulness to you. (Jeremiah 31:3 AMPC)

1. Our Heavenly Father loves us, and it has nothing to do with our performance or even how we act. In fact, Romans 8:38-39, says, "For I am convinced that neither death nor life, neither angels nor demons, neither the present nor the future, nor any powers, neither height nor depth, nor anything else in all creation, will be able to separate us from the love of God that is in Christ Jesus our Lord" (NIV).

   This may blow your mind, but even sin can't separate us from God's love. God loves us whether we are in sin or not. The reason He wants us out of sin is because sin opens the door for satan to come in and out of our lives. It has nothing to do with His love for us because everlasting means everlasting. Everlasting means unchanging.

2. Whether or not we received a promotion at work, were named employee of the month, was cast in the theater production, or got a scholarship, God accepts and encourages us. We may or may not have accomplished our goals this year, but it doesn't change God's love for us. Ephesians 1:3 says, "Praise be to the God and Father of our Lord Jesus Christ, who has blessed us in the heavenly realms with every spiritual blessing in Christ" (NIV). **God chose us before we were born so our acceptance has nothing to do with performance or achievements.**

3. God will never reject us. John 6:37 says, "However, those the Father has given me will come to me, and I will never reject them" (NLT).

›› ASK YOURSELF…

What have I built my foundation and security upon?

How have I handled rejection in the past?
What adjustments do I need to make?

Am I firmly rooted and grounded in God's love?
If not, what changes can I make?

A FINAL WORD OF ENCOURAGEMENT

YOU ARE NOT ALONE

Let us hold unswervingly to the hope we profess, for he who promised is faithful. And let us consider how we may spur one another on toward love and good deeds. Let us not give up meeting together, as some are in the habit of doing, but let us encourage one another — and all the more as you see the Day approaching. (Hebrews 10:23-25 NIV)

You are not alone. Jesus Christ promised to be with you always. God, maker of Heaven and Earth, the One who formed and knit you together in the womb will never leave nor forsake you. The Body of Christ, the Church, the Family of God gathers themselves together regularly to pray unceasing for, care for, minister to, serve, give to, and love one another.

You are not alone. The enemy of your soul seeks to isolate you, lie to you, steal from you, and ultimately kill you. His lie is that you are an orphan. Nevertheless, God in Christ Jesus has adopted you into His Family, the Church, and the Army of God to encourage you, equip you, educate you, and empower you in the Holy Spirit to destroy the works of the devil.

You are not alone. Christians together are a team accomplishing much for the Kingdom of God. Be bold and courageous. If God be for us, who can be against us? No one! We are more than conquerors through Christ who loves us and gave Himself for us.

You are not alone.

Get out of your closet, your cave, your pit of depression.
Leave your pity party, and your funk.
Forsake your critical, negative, cynical, attitude.
Don't listen to those naysayers around you.
Join ranks with the saints and destroy
the words and works of the enemy.
Be kind to one another.
Remember that you have the mind of Christ.
Pray not for what you want but for what God wants.
Love, forgive, encourage, empower, equip, and enlarge
the godly dreams and visions of others and when you do...
The enemies of your peace will flee. NEVER QUIT!
Do your part and let God do His part.
Together in Christ, WE WIN!

Now take a moment and preach to your spirit. This book isn't just for you, it's for everyone you know. You are to be an encourager. Speak and preach these Words of God to yourself as you share this book and minister encouragement to others. These are paraphrased just for you!

ENCOURAGEMENT CONFESSIONS

My mouth will encourage myself in the Lord and others; comfort from my lips will bring relief. (Job 16:5)

You hear, O Lord, the desire of the afflicted; you encourage them, and you listen to my cry. (Psalm 10:17)

I am committed to saying much to encourage and strengthen others. (Acts 15:32)

If it is encouraging, let me encourage; if it is contributing to the needs of others, let me give generously; if it is leadership, let me govern diligently; if it is showing mercy, let me do it cheerfully. (Romans 12:8)

Therefore, I will encourage each other with affirming words. (1 Thessalonians 4:18)

Therefore, I will encourage others and build others up continually. (1 Thessalonians 5:11)

I will encourage the hearts of others and strengthen them in every good deed and word. (2 Thessalonians 2:17)

GOOD MENTAL HEALTH CONFESSIONS AND PRAYER

I have the mind of Christ. (1 Corinthians 2:16)

Let the peace of God, which surpasses all understanding, guard my heart and my mind in Christ Jesus. (Philippians 4:7)

God has not given me a spirit of fear, but of power, love, and a sound mind. (2 Timothy 1:7)

I don't fear because you are with me. I am not dismayed because you are my God. You strengthen me and help me. (Isaiah 41:10).

My mind, will, and emotions find rest in God alone; my hope and salvation comes from Him. God is my rock and my fortress. (Psalm 62:1, 5-6)

I do not worry or feel anxious about anything; instead, I pray about everything continually thanking God along the way. (Philippians 4:6)

I am the righteousness of God in Christ Jesus. (2 Corinthians 5:21)

I am a winner. God always causes me to triumph in Him. (2 Corinthians 2:14)

I am not just a conqueror. I am MORE than a conqueror in Christ Jesus. (Romans 8:37)

No weapon formed against me (my mind) shall prosper. (Isaiah 54:17)

Father God,
Thank You for the truth of Your Word. You said that
You wish above all that I would prosper and be in
health even as my soul prospers. I receive that now
and on purpose I choose to cast down every negative
thought and replace it with the truth of Your Word.
In Jesus' Name, Amen.

Use this book as a practical tool as you navigate through your mental health journey. You no longer have to feel worried, rejected, discouraged, depressed, or stressed. God's will for you is good mental health. And you can have what you say, so claim it today!

PRAYER OF SALVATION

"For God so loved the world, that He gave His only begotten Son, that whosoever believeth in Him should not perish, but have everlasting life." (John 3:16 KJV)

God's Love: God loves you and He has a wonderful plan for your life.

God's Gift: To the world→ Jesus the Savior (His only begotten Son)

God's Reason: Because of Adam's disobedience all are born sinners and destined to the lake of fire. The Good News is God doesn't want you to go there. He sent Jesus in your place.

The Sinner's Response: You must believe this Good News and receive Jesus as the Lord and Ruler of your life.

Repent
Believe
Call
Confess

***** REPEAT THIS PRAYER OUT LOUD *****

Dear God,
*I **repent** of my sin.*
*I **believe** that Jesus died on the cross in my place and was raised from the dead for me.*
*I **call** on You, Jesus, and invite You now to come into my life.*
*I **confess** You as Lord of my life.*
Thank You, Father, for saving me.
In Jesus' name. Amen.

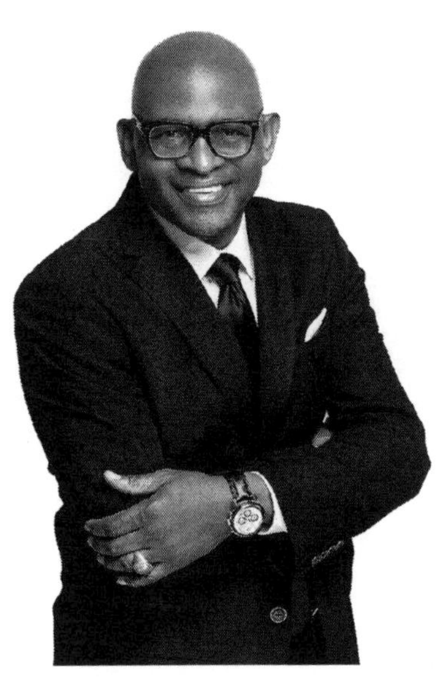

ABOUT THE AUTHOR

Mike Moore is the founder and CEO of Mike Moore Ministries and author of numerous books including the popular "Weep Not: Overcoming Grief, Disappointment, and Loss" and "Moving from Tragedy to Triumph" and "Muted Voice." He built this global ministry decades ago upon the simple yet profound truth that "The Word of God is the Answer" for every situation. His easy-to-follow messages provide practical ways to apply God's Word to everyday, real-life circumstances.

He is also the founding pastor of Faith Chapel. In addition to providing spiritual mentorship to an alliance of pastors, Moore can be seen on his Answers That Work television broadcast, YouTube channel, How To Win podcast, and at conferences.

He is married to Kennetha, and they have two adult children, Michael and Tiffany.

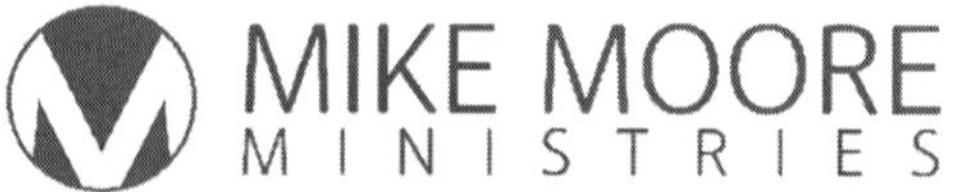

ABOUT MIKE MOORE MINISTRIES

Mike Moore Ministries, a global ministry founded by Mike Moore, was built upon the simple yet profound truth that "The Word of God is the Answer" to all of life's questions. Through various mediums which include television, digital, and print, Moore teaches that God wants His people to live a prosperous life— a prosperity that exceeds the boundaries of just finances. This prosperity encompasses spiritual prosperity, physical health, relationships, mental health, and financial independence.

Additional resources can be obtained by visiting mikemoore.com or by calling toll-free 1-866-930-WORD (9673).

Healing Is for All
Mike Moore

Is divine healing for everybody in the body of Christ? Is it God's will for all His children to be healthy and free from sickness? Is it God's will to heal only some and leave others sick or in pain for His glory or to develop their character? The greatest barrier to the faith of many seeking healing is the uncertainty in our minds as to whether it is the will of God to heal all. Nearly everyone knows that God is able to heal and that He does heal some, but there is much in modern beliefs that keep people from knowing what the Bible really teaches – that *Healing Is for All*. Healing and health are available to you right now!

ISBN: 978-1-7333716-0-5
4"x6" paperback
ORDER TODAY at mikemoore.com

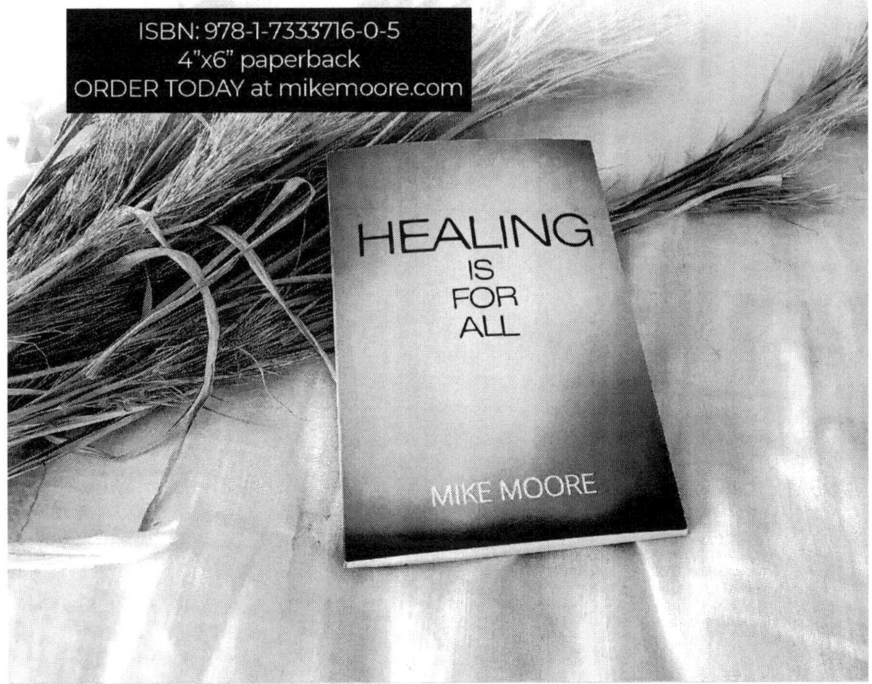

ENEMIES TO PEACE

Reclaim your mental health and discover your inner peace with these audio lessons by Mike Moore. Choose from these six series.

- Enemies to Peace: Depression (2-part series)
- Enemies to Peace: Discouragement (2-part series)
- Enemies to Peace: Rejection (3-part series)
- Enemies to Peace: Stress (3-part series)
- Enemies to Peace: Suicide (1-part series)
- Enemies to Peace: Worry (6-part series)

These enemies go against what God desires for your life. Start your healing journey now by visiting www.mikemoore.com and searching for *Enemies to Peace*.